Therapeutic Communication

Tova Navarra, BA, RN
Myron A. Lipkowitz, RP, MD
John G. Navarra, Jr., Esq., JD

SLACK Incorporated, 6900 Grove Road, Thorofare, New Jersey 08086

Printed in the United States of America

Library of Congress Catalog Card Number: 88-43159

ISBN: 1-55642-075-7

Published by: SLACK Incorporated
               6900 Grove Road
               Thorofare, NJ 08086-9447

Last digit is print number: 10   9   8   7   6   5

May We meet our responsibility to learn to get along with each other, to learn to care for one another, and to show it.

—*Thomas W. Muldary,*
Interpersonal Relations for Health Professionals

All are masked sometimes with silence, arrogance, anger. Thus we cannot judge the package by its wrappings...we can only accept the contents as having value.

—*Peter Seymour*, I Am My Brother

But separating himself farther and farther from the animal, man conceived the desire for a sympathetic environment and he invented words to express his grief, in order not to be alone in the realization of it.

Xanthes, Speech, How to Use Effectively

DEDICATION

For Celeste Scala Roberts, whose caring communication makes everything better, and Rose E. Treihart, who has been a stellar role model for health professionals for the past 40 years.

—T.N. and J.G.N.

In loving memory of my parents: Irving Lipkowitz, who taught by example the meaning of love of mankind and civil rights, and Rena Wineberg Lipkowitz, whose inspiration and loving encouragement were always there when I needed them. And to my wife, Jill, for her love, tolerance, and support.

—M.A.L.

Contents

ACKNOWLEDGMENTS

The authors wish to thank Yolanda T. Navarra for encouraging comments and typing services; physicians and rehabilitation staff at Kimball Medical Center, Lakewood, N.J., and staff members at Garden State Rehabilitation Hospital, Toms River, N.J.; Warren Deutsch, Ed.D.; Thomas Bartolino, PT; Donna Ziarkowski, PT; Andy Ford; Priscilla Loughner; patients who freely shared their experiences; our illustrator, Ed Gabel, whose delightful drawings add humor and humanity to the book, and Harry Benson and Stephanie Scanlon of Slack, Inc., who championed this project.

We also acknowledge each other for the wonderful rapport maintained through every stage of authorship, including the stress.

PREFACE

NON-THERAPEUTIC WORDS ARE US

If you reflect on how people actually talk to each other on a daily basis, you'll hear a rash of non-therapeutic communication. Let's put the health-professional role aside for a moment and visualize working in a large corporation. No one is a "patient"; everyone is busy, and a lot of interaction goes on among the employees in order for them to get their work done and their deadlines met.

During a typical day at a major daily newspaper headquarters, for example, communication readily takes on many of these characteristics:

—small talk
—gossip
—sarcastic or critical remarks
—commiseration
—humor
—"shop" talk
—acknowledgment
—confidential exchanges
—compliments
—no response

At home, communication may be less restricted than it is in the workplace. Family members unrestrainedly fly off the handle, criticize, call each other names, and make fun of each other. Somehow, all is forgiven and the family endures. It just seems natural to say what you have to say without guard, and you'd think it unnatural to have to ponder another's every pause and gesture and give a "trained" response.

In short, we traumatize each other far more frequently than we consciously try to be therapeutic. Which is why therapeutic communication techniques have been devised. As psychology developed as an important branch of the health-care professions, people began to recognize what questions and statements encouraged or discouraged the patient. It became apparent that certain techniques drew more insightful information than others, and through these insights, patients had a better chance of resolving their conflicts. Psychologists and other counselors through the decades charted the techniques and included them in their formal courses of study.

Somehow, other health-related professions become bogged down in huge curricula, and how to communicate with patients seems a

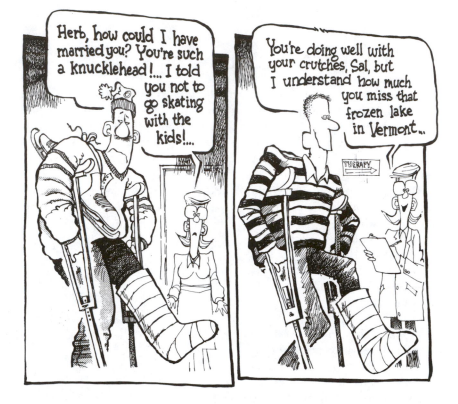

small fraction of it. While programs are ever-changing, many dentists, physicians, nurses, and various therapists reported they received little, if any, training in therapeutic communication.

Why give such a pivotal part of your career short shrift?

This book is not about physical or occupational therapy techniques. It offers communication techniques that any health professional can use. And if you think communication is just a matter of common sense, think again. In fact, most of our instinctive responses—things we say throughout the day to each other—are often non-therapeutic. For example, did you know that asking a patient "Why? . . ." is usually threatening? Did you think telling a depressed patient, "We all suffer sometimes" discounts his feelings even if you're trying to be warm and sincere and helpful? Until you're aware of how you sound and the implications of what you're saying, you really don't "just know" how to be therapeutic.

Until you become accustomed to hearing "buzz" words that are your cue for using one technique or another, slip this book in your lab-coat pocket and refer to it whenever you wish. It's meant to be "user-friendly." And its purpose is not to take over your individual approach to your challenges as a therapist, but to give you a little push in the right direction.

We're advocating awareness as the initial tool. Just as a singer can't sing well unless he hears himself with a sensitive ear, a therapist (or any health professional) can't just start talking and hope the patient survives. Because communicating well is a skill that requires practice, we offer some insights and techniques which will help make your words as healing as your physical or occupational treatments.

About the Authors

Tova Navarra, a registered nurse and magna cum laude graduate of Seton Hall University, is the author of the internationally syndicated column, "Your Body." A staff writer at The Asbury Park Press, Ms. Navarra has also written *Playing It Smart: What to Do When You're on Your Own*, published by Barron's Educational Series, Inc.; *The New Jersey Shore: A Vanishing Splendor; Jim Gary: His Life and Art*; and *Your Body: Highlights of the Human Anatomy*. She also illustrated *Drugs and Man* (Doubleday & Co.) and has contributed photographs and illustrations to numerous books, newspapers and magazines.

The author of articles in *Today's OR Nurse, RN, Today's Student PT* and other professional journals, Ms. Navarra is a contributing editor to the *American Journal of Nursing*. She also has worked as a charge nurse at an intermediate-care facility for psychiatric patients.

Myron A. Lipkowitz received a BS in pharmacy from Duquesne University in 1961 and worked for ten years as a retail pharmacist. He earned his MD from the Universidad Autonoma de Guadalajara in Mexico. After completing two years of post-graduate training at St. Joseph's Hospital and Medical Center in Paterson, NJ, he worked for two years in Uniontown, PA as an emergency room physician and maintained a rural family practice in the mountain community of Markleysberg. A family practitioner and allergist, he now shares a Howell, NJ office with his brother, Dr. Kenneth P. Lipkowitz, an internist.

Dr. Lipkowitz has two children, Kara and Michael, three step-children, Pamela, Kathleen and Christopher Campbell, and resides in Howell with his wife, Jill.

John Gabriel Navarra, Jr. is former Director of Legal Services at The New Jersey Council of Savings Institutions. Currently a solo law practitioner and formerly a teacher of physics and chemistry at Christian Brothers Academy, Mr. Navarra holds baccalaureate and master's degrees from Columbia College, Columbia University, and a master of arts in teaching and a juris doctor degree from Seton Hall University. He taught law, physics and German at Seton Hall Preparatory School for ten years. He is now working on a book of short stories.

Tova and John Navarra live in Monmouth County with their son John, a student at The Monmouth Conservatory of Music. Their daughter, Yolanda, is a staff writer at The Asbury Park Press.

About the Illustrator

Ed Gabel, raised in Port Clinton, Ohio, is the son of Thomas E. and Miriam E. Gabel. He began his art career under the direction of Jeanie Radloff at Port Clinton High School. After earning a B S degree in business administration from Miami University, in Oxford, Ohio, Mr. Gabel chose to pursue a career in cartooning and illustration. He works for *The Blade*, a Toledo newspaper, and is the illustrator of the internationally syndicated column, "Your Body."

CHAPTER I

Why Talk

Tova Navarra, BA, RN

"I said it in Hebrew—I said it in Dutch—
I said it in German and Greek:
But I wholly forgot (and it vexes me much)
That English is what you speak!"

—from *The Hunting of the Snark*
by Lewis Carroll

When ill or recovering from illness, some people talk a great deal, some talk some, and some not at all. Which category best describes you, the health care professional? How do you react to pain? What comforts you most when your body is out of whack? When you need to heal, who really speaks your language?

Student physical and occupational therapists, like other members of the health care team, have to learn a special "language" that allows them to speak effectively to just about anyone from Planet Earth. It is along the lines of Esperanto, but it doesn't require foreign sounds, changes in grammar or translations. Rather, it's a universal way to communicate with patients and it's based largely on a commonly used phrase—reading the "signals."

You can learn to assess a patient quickly by reading his or her signals—facial expression, body language, verbal responses—and gearing your manner toward the patient's needs. To a journalist, a key premise is: "Think of your poor reader." Similarly, to a therapist it is: "Think of your poor patient." Essentially, this means you should try to put yourself in the patient's position and see yourself objectively as a health caregiver. Just as the journalist wants his or her story to be informative, clear and maybe even entertaining, so should the therapist strive to give the patient information, positive therapy sessions, and maybe even a good deal of comforting and encouragement.

This usually involves conversation. Can you imagine a therapy session in which both the patient and the therapist are comatose? Nothing very therapeutic would come of that. Eventually, you will have to converse, and as the therapist, you are responsible for engineering the patient's cooperation to ensure that he or she reaches optimum functional level, if not full recovery. Physical therapy is not just expending energy; occupational therapy is not just conserving it. Both therapists rely heavily on how they get along and talk with their patients. You cannot compartmentalize a patient's physical and psychological needs. A patient isn't "the hip replacement in Room 314" or "the head trauma in 701." For any health caregiver, the patient is always the whole person, a body complete with personality and sensitivities: Mr. Jones, Mrs. Abel, Harry, or Mary or Jennifer.

This book is meant to guide you in developing your own style of therapeutic communication, but it's not limited only to interaction with your patients. At times, a little "tender loving care" goes a long way with a member of the patients' family or one of your professional colleagues, or, in fact, anyone with whom you exchange words. Think of how you communicate with your patient, classmate, teacher, spouse, or friend. The Golden Rule—treating others the way you want to be treated—is more golden than ever when it comes to health care.

Employing the Golden Rule requires that you consider your reasons for going into a therapeutic field. "I want to help people" rings through the halls of medical, nursing, physical therapy (PT), occupational therapy (OT), social work and other schools. Sister Elizabeth Kenny, one of the founders of physical therapy as we know it today, undoubtedly said it when she realized the need for reteaching motor coordination to polio victims. Wanting to help is a noble start and no one can find fault with it. But there is no substitute for acquiring a body of knowledge and then learning the most effective methods of using it. You have often heard people refer scornfully to "book learning" when they think a person has command of the theories, but that his or her practice of them is stiff or shaky.

A large part of successful professional practice is practice. Actors provide a good example here. Because they are beleaguered by the press and repeatedly asked the same questions, actors often compose stock answers to satisfy the reporters. The late Cary Grant was often asked how he developed his elegant image, and he would reply that he chose an elegant role model and worked on thinking and being elegant until he was. Actress Virginia Mayo, popular in the 1940s, had a stock response to flirtatious compliments on her shapely legs. "Thanks," Miss Mayo would say, "they get me around."[6]

Stock answers also help celebrities avoid saying something awkward on impulse. Using a stock answer, especially an amusing one, may help someone appear polished and confident.

There is no reason for health care professionals not to have a few stock phrases prepared in anticipation of an awkward or difficult situation. One pediatrician tried to help a young mother be more relaxed about her baby's first cold by saying to her, "It will last 14 days with the medicine and 2 weeks without it." His overall kind and competent manner gave the woman "permission" to smile while assuring her the baby would survive nicely. He did not rehearse it, but he used it when appropriate with anxious parents. As long as the health professional does not come across as flip or insensitive, some funny stock lines can ease many a tense encounter.

Don't worry if you're not a born comedian, however. We are not targeting the extremes. A therapist is only human and should realize everyone else is, too.

Those who have lost some autonomy as a result of disease or injury need to be reminded often that "they're only human" and that rehabilitation takes time. Patients who tend to be impatient may make it harder for themselves to recover. Other human characteristics a patient may exhibit include: anger, denial, fear, depression and helplessness. The therapist must assess and contend with whatever attitude the patient displays. The rehabilitative process is not easy, and it's probably safe to say it cannot go fast enough for the patient.

If psychological factors are in a patient's favor, rehabilitation has a better chance of progressing with a minimum of obstacles or setbacks. Dr. Howard Rusk, who developed a rehabilitation program for convalescent soldiers in the mid-1900s, said, "It's not enough to heal a man's physical wounds. You also have to heal his emotional wounds."[4]

To be honest, it's often harder work to deal with the soul than the body. Questions will arise, such as: What are we, mind readers? Does a license to practice PT or OT come with a crystal ball? What do patients want, anyway?

How many times you will ask yourself these questions! Brace yourself for that discouraged, "I'm-banging-my-head-against-a-brick-wall" feeling; it happens all the time in health care. Anticipate days when your patients will not want to see you or go through your regimen.

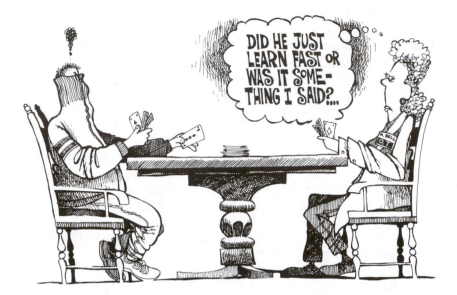

Just as you inform a patient in advance about any procedures so he or she won't feel coldly manipulated like a sack of potatoes, also inform yourself that there will be slumps. John Lennon's song lyric, "Nobody told me there'd be days like these," should not apply to health care personnel.

Fortunately, the positive side of your career choice comes through regularly enough for you to feel your work is valued and effective and worth getting up for in the morning. This holds true in many professions.

During a grueling job interview, a prospective young teacher was asked how he would handle several thorny situations with students. The interviewee remained level-headed and answered every question as sincerely and intelligently as he could. The interviewer finally challenged him by asking, "And what if all those methods fail?"

"Then I've failed," the young man replied.

He got the job. The interviewer decided his realistic viewpoint would help the new teacher cope with a school full of teenaged boys. It also suggested the teacher did not need to think of himself as "super-teacher," but rather as a competent professional willing to learn from experience.

You do not have to be "super-therapist," either. Pleading or expecting perfection sets you up for disillusionment. Why be so hard on yourself when you'll be telling your patients not to worry if they progress slowly? Sometimes we forget to apply the advice we give patients to ourselves. The professional, no matter how gifted or experienced, has to frequently examine his or her modus operandi, make an assessment, and evaluate it the same way he or she would evaluate a patient's chart.

The "practice what you preach" principle is not easy, but a minimal effort may bring surprising results. In short, as you communicate therapeutically with your patients, communicate therapeutically with yourself. Dr. David Viscott, a California psychiatrist and best-selling author, called the technique "being a good parent to yourself." Think how encouraging and compassionate most parents would be toward a disappointed child, and project that image in your own mind when you need it.

The concept of good parenting can work in many cases, but, particularly when used in conjunction with patients, the professional has to guard against its backfiring. As a therapist, you are in a position to become a kind of guru to a patient. When he or she considers his or her therapy an exhilarating experience, the patient may put you on a pedestal right up there with the vision of recovery. Your supportive manner and interest in the patient's well-being should not allow you to become a surrogate parent, son, daughter or best friend. Convey your interest with an unflagging, realistic approach.

In his book, *Making People Talk*, talk-show host Barry Farber advises that you try to find something to talk about, keeping the other person's interests in mind. You can always discuss the therapeutic treatment or the patient's progress, but you can get on a more personal, "feeling" level without invading privacy. Farber wrote, "Don't ask Linda (who acts and paints) what role she's played (if she's not well-known)—ask *about* acting. Ask what inspires her to paint."[5]

Farber's rule here is to make sure your questions are real. How to ask "real" questions will be explored later on in this book.

The reality is that the therapist must also be persuasive at times. A discouraged, angry or tired patient needs a bit of cheerleading and a firm advocate in you. Persuasiveness involves not only what you say, but how you say it.

Writer Philip Lesly used a premise of Aristotle's in his book, *How We Discommunicate*: "It is not enough to know *what* we ought to say; we must also say it *as* we ought; much help is thus afforded toward producing the right impression of a speech."[7]

Lesly included the idea of tugging at a common thread, which applies as naturally to a speaker and his or her audience as it does to a therapist and his or her patient. In being persuasive lies "the ability to find the audience's sensitive nerve and to connect one's ideas with it. . . . Part of it is chemistry, part of it is sincerity, part of it is sensing how to stand in another's psyche long enough to fine tune it."[8]

In order to do this, Lesly proposed a "cure" for discommunication: "Acknowledge your mistakes, be open to ideas and ask questions, find out what skillful communicators would teach you, and note how you read, speak, write and use body language."[9]

When a patient acted ornery (yes, some are downright obnoxious!) or less than enthusiastic, one physical therapist used a gesture she learned from her five-year-old niece Anna. Instead of holding up a straight forefinger in reprimand, the way Mom or a teacher might do, Anna made a hook of her index finger like Walt Disney's wicked witch and simultaneously struck a menacing facial expression. The family howled when Anna tried this on her grandmother, who had told her to go to bed.

The PT recounted this story to a patient who refused to move out of bed into a wheelchair. The therapist then crooked her finger at the patient and put on a wicked face, and the patient, a grandmother herself, broke into laughter as she made the transfer. The therapist hoped her patient would stay in good spirits through her physical therapy session and was grateful for reaching a mutually agreeable topic—children—with her patient.

Finding a patient's "sensitive nerve" may be difficult. In domestic situations, a dialogue might unfold as follows:

> HUSBAND: What's the matter?
> WIFE: Nothing.

The husband here knows very well there's trouble brewing, however, just by his wife's body language or the tone of her voice.

A similar type of dialogue often arises between parents and their teenaged children:

> PARENT: Where did you go?
> TEEN: Out.
> PARENT: What did you do?
> TEEN: Nothing.

The teenager protects his privacy, just as a patient may withhold information from the therapist. It is important that the therapist recognize the delicate border that exists between ideal communication, consisting of an exchange of information, and those things that are rightfully private.

Communicating with another person is taking a risk. Think about all the risks you take each day as you interact with your patients, their family members and your fellow professionals. In our society, it may be risky to tell the truth when someone asks, "How are you?" because she may not really be interested in anything more than a quick greeting. You are taking a risk when you make the commitment to become a health care student, when you show up for your clinical rotation no matter how you feel, when you accept the responsibility of helping an injured person heal. You are risking something every time you start a conversation with a patient or discuss a problem with your supervisor. But do not misunderstand. Communicating does not have to be like walking the plank. The risks are reasonable when you've learned some therapeutic communication techniques. These don't ensure you'll never make a mistake, but they may help you recover well from one and avoid others in the future. They also do not preclude your using your own best judgment or gut instinct to deal with a situation. The philosopher Elbert Hubbard gave us a memorable line about this: "To avoid criticism, do nothing, say nothing, be nothing." If you care about something, your caring will be communicated even if someone else criticizes your words or actions.

In an *American Journal of Nursing* article entitled "Caring Comes First," the authors explore the risks—stress, vulnerability and burnout—of developing a therapist-client relationship.

"Caring enables people to discern problems, to recognize possible solutions, *and* to implement those solutions. Caring makes the nurse notice which interventions help, causes the nurse to notice subtle signs of patient improvement or deterioration. . . . Caring is primary because it sets up the condition of trust where help can be given and help can be received. This is why nursing can never be reduced to mere technique."[1]

This applies well to physical and occupational therapists and other professionals. Whether you care or not, and how you utilize your caring, are at the core of therapeutic communication. Your willingness to work with patients affects what you say and all the nuances of it.

The same article also points out that it's important to achieve the right level of interaction with patients, which may actually be what an eager-to-please therapist thinks of as doing too little. But "(i)t takes courage to be involved and to offer what you can even though it may not be enough."[2]

While a small contribution can go a long way, health care professionals tend to put down their efforts because they feel inexperienced or insecure. Helen Keller, the blind and deaf woman who owed her ability to experience a cultured life to an inexperienced therapist, once said, "Security is mostly a superstition. It does not exist in nature, nor do the children of men as a whole experience it. Avoiding danger is no safer in the long run than outright exposure. Life is either a daring adventure or nothing."[11]

Your education, good intentions and a little nerve can cushion some of the risks, however. Anatomy and physiology class teaches you about Broca's area of the brain, which enables you to translate your thoughts into speech. Add to that information the old proverb, "Think first, then speak," and you have a powerful tool.

The ancient Roman philosopher Seneca said we must feel what we speak before we can speak what we feel, which takes the concept of thinking first to a deeper level. For you as the therapist, feeling first may best be employed in the patient's, not necessarily your own, favor. The feeling is consistent compassion for those who require rehabilitative services. How can you acquaint yourself more deliberately with this feeling? Try reversed-role sessions with your classmates or facility personnel. For example, imagine you had been in a car accident that forced your head into the windshield. You suffered head injuries that truncated your former lifestyle. Make a list of things you used to do—go to college, enjoy dates, take care of yourself, hold a job. Make a list of things you can't do now—speak clearly, coordinate your muscles, remember past events, retain what you study. Really envision being this patient with his or her deficits. Have a classmate play the part of therapist and try for an Academy Award in making the situation realistic. You could be amazed at the result. What you say to each other in role-playing is often very humanly universal and you can learn much from the encounter.

Linda S. Dean, director of The National Training Center for Rehabilitation Hospital Services Corporation (the country's largest provider of physical rehabilitation services in Dallas, Texas), spoke of intraprofessional role-reversal. She called it "mock-staffing," in which the rehab professionals "switched" roles to gather insights into how they could most effectively work together for the good of the patients.

"We'd been having problems with appropriate communication not only with patients and their families, but with each other," Ms. Dean said. "For example, PTs and OTs were using jargon and misunderstanding each other. Some people think jargon is power, but saying words people don't understand leads to disharmony at times. The mock-staffing really works. Staff members 'playing' each other laughed a lot and spit out words they'd heard but didn't understand. It's a nonthreatening way to solve problems of frustration and embarrassment among professionals."

Ms. Dean added that the mock-staffing can be especially valuable in a facility where there is a frequent turnover of staff. Because people ideally have to pull together, the session increased the team members' awareness of how they need to explain things to others. The logical next step after communicating better among themselves is communicating better with patients. Ms. Dean believes the biggest communication problem therapists have with patients is how to get them internally motivated for the difficult, tedious tasks toward wellness ahead of them. "There's a lack of understanding on the patients' part of the amount of motivation they have to get better," she said. "They think, 'the doctor or the PT will cure me.' But it's a long, hard road and they have to be willing to work, especially long-term patients who become depressed, progress very slowly, or, say, the spinal-cord injured whose fourth- to sixth-grade reading comprehension level affects their ability to understand [professional vocabulary].

"Bringing things down to simpler terms can be hard for educated members of the rehab team," Ms. Dean said.

A poem called "The Centipede" was included in the text of a 1950s elementary school book. Physical and occupational therapists would get the greatest kick out of it, because it describes a little, 100-legged insect who was asked by a frog, "Which leg comes after which?"

The frog's question started the centipede thinking for the first time about the mechanics of walking. She was baffled to distraction and for a while was unable to move at all. Consider how you might strain for an analytical explanation of things you do automatically, either through practice or reflex. What if a Martian landed and asked you to explain how you digest your food, or how your blood circulates or how you drive?

As a professional talking with your patients, you may realize the multi-tiered dynamics occurring simultaneously, but don't let your awareness of each segment inhibit the overall flow of things. Certainly, don't let it stop you from freely initiating communication.

Elizabeth, an elderly schizophrenic patient in a geriatric/psychiatric facility, never smiled or made discernible eye contact with anyone. Her eyes appeared glassy and staring; her mouth was always slightly open, but she remained silent. As she plodded down the hall, Elizabeth held her tremorous hands up in front of her. Actually, she might be frightening-looking to many people. One afternoon, she went to the nurses' station for her medication, which included an antibiotic prescribed for a respiratory infection. Accustomed to Elizabeth's reticence, the nurse said to her, "Well, you look a little better today. You must feel better."

"To a certain extent," Elizabeth replied.

The nurse almost fell over to hear a verbal response. Not only did

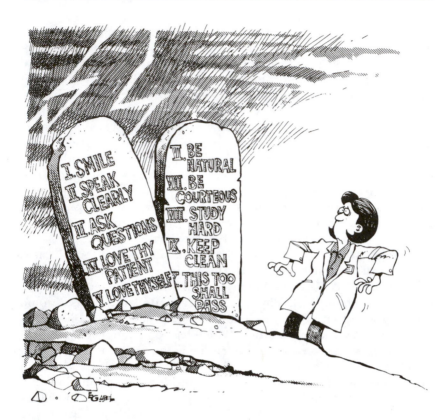

she not expect one, she had often wondered if Elizabeth was *able* to speak.

The story of Elizabeth and the nurse illustrates the need to risk communicating, even if that need lies tucked away in some remote ward of a person's mind. In their book *You & Media: Mass Communication and Society*, authors David G. Clark and William B. Blankenburg expressed what it means to lose communication.

"It's as true for modern man as it was for his primal ancestors: losing communication is a kind of dying, and that's why we shun the loss. . . . The severest punishment society can impose upon a deviant person is complete sensory deprivation: the death sentence. Scarcely less severe are solitary confinement, banishment, and ostracism. The strongest sanction of the Roman Catholic Church is—note the word— excommunication."[3]

The Bible story of the Tower of Babel brings to the fore another message about obstacles in communication. The people of Mesopotamia, descendants of Noah, wanted to build a tower that would reach into heaven and they set to work on it. God disapproved of such a tower, however, and caused the workers to speak different languages. One scientific theory is that the tower, a Ziggurat structure, created echoes that badly distorted the workers' calls to each other. In any case, the end to their communication meant the end of their project.

The following chapters were written for "team players" who wish to function more smoothly and happily as an enduring team. Don't forget that teams are made up of individuals. Communication is our link to sharing our individuality, learning, teaching, symbiosis, even relaxation and pain reduction. Your capacity for understanding yourself and others successfully comes through choosing your words and gestures well.

In so choosing, remember the bones. This is the story of an old Irishman giving advice to a young man. "Now, Michael," he said, "just remember the three bones and you'll be fine—the wishbone to keep you going after things, the jawbone to help you ask the questions necessary to find them, and the backbone to keep you at it until you get them."[10]

References

1. Benner, P. and Wrubel, J. "Caring Comes First." *American Journal of Nursing*, August 1988: 1073-75.
2. Benner, P. and Wrubel, J. "Caring Comes First." *American Journal of Nursing*, August 1988: 1073-75.
3. Clark, D.G. *You and Media: Mass Communication and Society*, San Francisco: Cornfield Press, 1973.
4. Darby, P. *Your Career in Physical Therapy*. Englewood, N.J.: Julia Messner, a Division of Simon & Schuster, 1969.
5. Farber, B. *Making People Talk*. New York: Morrow & Co., Inc., 1987.
6. King, E. *Glorify Yourself*. New York: Prentice Hall, Inc., 1942.
7. Lesly, P. *How We Discommunicate*. New York: AMACOM, A Division of American Management Associations, 1979.
8. Lesly, P. *How We Discommunicate*. New York: AMACOM, A Division of American Management Associations, 1979.
9. Lesly, P. *How We Discommunicate*. New York: AMACOM, A Division of American Management Associations, 1979.
10. *Remember the Bones*. Los Angeles: Science of Mind Publications, 1988.
11. *Step to the Edge and Fly!* Los Angeles: Science of Mind Publications, 1988.

Exercises

Questions for discussion and situations for role-playing:
Introduction: In role-playing exercises, students may conceive of
many different scenarios. The more students can draw on their clinical and other experience to supply realistic detail and put themselves
in the places of patients and therapists, the more meaningful the
exercises will be. Scripts may be adlibbed or written out with directions such as physical setting, body language, facial expression, and
so on. Students are encouraged to act out situations fraught with
significant conflict. Even if students are not sure at first how to resolve
the conflicts in a professional manner, the exercises will serve to
sensitize them to their patients and make them more experienced
and confident. Group discussion and the instructor's advice will help
lead the students closer to a good resolution of the problems they
pose.

1. a. Do you talk a lot, some or hardly at all, if you're given a
      choice?
   b. Were you encouraged by parents, teachers and others to
      speak up or hold back?
   c. Do you remember specific instances when your attempts to
      speak up were rewarded and encouraged or met with disap-
      pointment and discouraged?
2. Describe a specific instance, professional or personal, in which
   you might have communicated your needs better. What did you
   say? What was the response? How might you have taken the
   interaction further through more effective communication?
3. How do you and your family members communicate your pain?
   Do you suffer in silence? Do you view suffering in silence as a
   virtue? How do you react when others communicate their pain
   and problems to you? Do you pull back? Is your sympathy
   aroused?
4. Let one student play the role of a patient who has recently had
   a hip replaced and is now in pain. This patient shows her pain
   by her facial expressions and body language, by *few* if any words,
   and seems to be pushing the therapist to the threshold of her
   frustration. The therapist persists in trying to find out just what
   the problem is.
5. A student playing a patient seems to be half trying and half
   listening to the instruction of another student playing an OT.
   The patient expresses frustration and an "I-can-never-get-this"
   attitude. The students interact and react.

6. What risks does a therapist take in practicing his or her profession? Are these risks frightening? Are the risks part of the challenge and excitement of the profession?
7. One student is playing the role of a young patient who has suffered head injuries that truncated his former lifestyle. He used to go to college, date often and hold a job. Now he cannot speak clearly, coordinate his muscles, remember past events or retain what he studies. Another student-therapist is trying to motivate him.

Study Questions

1. Stock answers
   a) should never be used because they show a reluctance to confront the patient in a personal way
   b) may help deal with awkward or difficult situations as long as they don't come across as flip or insensitive
2. A therapist must deal
   a) with physical problems only
   b) with both physical and emotional problems
3. A health care professional _____ become a surrogate parent or best friend.
   a) should
   b) should not
4. Good communication _____ involves risk-taking.
   a) sometimes
   b) never
5. Which of these should you consider when speaking to a patient?
   a) what the patient says
   b) how he says it
   c) the patient's body language
   d) all of these
6. Jargon
   a) is power
   b) may lead to misunderstanding and disharmony
7. Mock-staffing is
   a) usually not worthwhile because it is so difficult to imagine the feelings of patients
   b) a nonthreatening way to solve problems of frustration and embarrassment among professionals
8. In communicating with patients to motivate them for difficult and tedious tasks, you must overcome their erroneous notion that

a) they will be primarily passive and the doctor or PT will cure them
b) they will be active and primarily responsible for their progress

CHAPTER II

Communication Techniques: Conversational Examples

Tova Navarra, BA, RN

When Shakespeare wrote "All the world's a stage and all the men and women merely players," he was correct. Not only are we players, but each of us comes equipped with his or her own book of lines and directions about how the play should go.

Think of any director! How is he or she going to get people to stick to the same subject, listen efficiently enough to react to what was *really* said instead of what they wanted to hear, resolve the play's main conflicts, and keep an audience in the house?

An article in the January 9, 1989 issue of *Newsweek* highlighted communication pitfalls, such as clashing views, withheld information and missed signals.[1] Although it focused on the conventional mish-mash that married couples often fall into, the article can be applied to anyone who has to work as a director in any sense. In your case, as therapist, your "theater" is created by a hospital, rehab facility, private offices or people's homes. Your cast? The young, old, middle-aged, sweet, testy, smart, ignorant, refined, vulgar, compliant, difficult, the healthy and the chronically ill. In short, you've got to be ready for just about anything. As one veteran manager put it as he gestured toward an office full of busy people, "Everyone here is a story."

R. Jeffrey Coley, chief kinesiologist and physical therapist at the Veterans Administration Medical Center in East Orange, N.J., said nothing is foolproof, but therapists should remember: You're there to treat the whole patient, not just the personality.

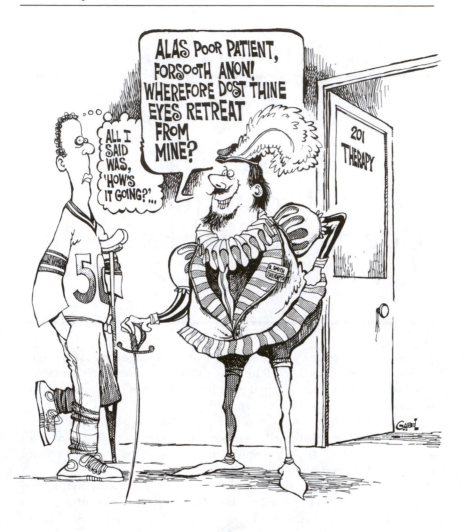

"It all depends on the patient," Coley said. "Some are mean as a whistle, some are easy to get along with. There's always the one or two patients you feel some friction with, but it's the professional's job to deal with controversy and treat the patient in a professional manner.

"The patient needs to be enthusiastic about his treatment," Coley added. "Some outpatients come in to chat even though they could get a hot pack at home. If you take that personal approach—not a factory or production line [attitude]—and delve into a patient's life a little bit to show concern for his well-being, he'll be more receptive to the therapy."

Coley became a physical therapist after working in several other fields that did not suit him.

"The first time I saw a quadriplegic and saw his head on the pillow, I thought about how he couldn't go to the bathroom, that he'd be confined to an institution for the rest of his life," Coley said. "I decided to help in spite of what kind of care he needed.

"Others had shunned him. A lot of people can't stand their field, and you can see it in how they treat patients. But when you can pick up a guy who's stroked out, aphasic, can't care for himself, and he starts to respond . . .

"When his wife comes to you and says he can use his trapeze and transfer board, or he started walking in the parallel bars . . .

"When you see slow progress toward ADL (activities of daily living) and see a smile on the patient's face . . .

"When an amputee can walk without a cane . . .

"When they come back a year later and say, 'Hi, Jeff,'—then you know you're in the right field."

The following pages deal with many "stories" and how conversations between therapist and patient develop. Each is a "play" with realistic situations and emotions; each is an example of a technique you can use if you find yourself in a similar encounter.

Introducing Yourself

"The Informer"

> THERAPIST: Hello, Mrs. Hamilton. My name is Sandra Jackson. I'm a physical therapist and this morning I'll be doing some exercises with you to help you strengthen your arms. (she smiles)
> PATIENT: Oh, hello. Nice to meet you, Miss Jackson. It's good to know there's hope for these old limbs. I want to do everything I can to work with you. It sure would be great if I could hold my new grandson in my arms. (she smiles)
> THERAPIST: A new grandson! How wonderful! Let's really set that goal. The exercises you'll be doing may seem difficult at first, but we can start slowly and work our way up.
> PATIENT: My mother always said, "Little by little." You're such a pleasant young lady. I don't think I'll have much trouble having you for a physical therapist. You know, before my operation, I used to . . .

And they're off. All first encounters should be so easy! What is illustrated here is a therapist's introduction of herself to the patient. She greeted the patient formally by name. She stated her whole name, her title and her purpose for the session. She smiled.

It is your responsibility to offer your patients this information and see to it they absorb it.

In this scene, the patient couldn't have been more congenial and accepting of the therapist. She's the kind of patient who spoils health professionals. And she has contributed to "The Informer" technique because she offered information to the therapist—a positive return.

Here is another version of "The Informer."

> THERAPIST: Hi. I'm Rudy. How 'bout if you get started by putting your arms up. (patient starts to comply) That's it, put 'em way up over your head (patient winces in pain, still compliant) and down. OK. Not bad.
> PATIENT: I hate to sound ignorant, but may I ask you what all that was about?
> THERAPIST: Oh, sure, Mrs. H. It's your physical therapy.
> PATIENT: Oh, yes. My doctor mentioned I'd need physical therapy. Are you a therapist?
> THERAPIST: (winks at her) Who'd ya think?
> PATIENT: Well, I just wanted to make sure . . .
> THERAPIST: Not to worry, love. I'm official. Anyhow, tell me about your operation . . .

Whew! This therapist almost ruined his chances with the patient, but he finally started down the right track when he asked her for information about her condition. Sweet Mrs. Hamilton! She was more "The Informer" this time. Luckily, she was able to ask questions. And she *wants* to have a pleasant rapport with her caregivers, so she's willing to give even this casual young man the leeway his personality seems to require. His role as "The Informer" needs a lot more work, however. The next patient may not have Mrs. Hamilton's nurturing disposition, as follows:

> PATIENT: What the hell do you *want*? Why can't everyone leave me alone?
> THERAPIST: Good morning, Mr. Peterson. I'm Sandra Jackson, a physical therapist . . .
> PATIENT: Aw, geez! You gonna make me get on that lousy bike like the other girl made me do? Well, I'm not interested right now.

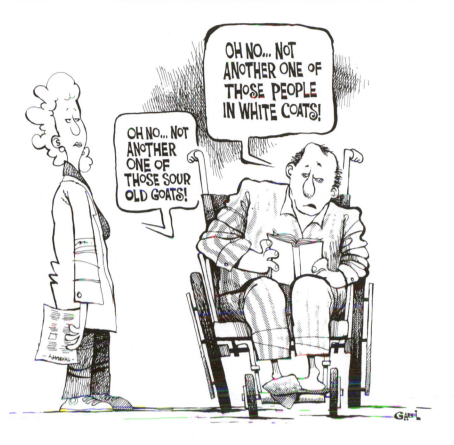

THERAPIST: Mr. Peterson, I'm Sandra Jackson, your physical therapist. I'd like to talk to you about your angina and your physical therapy ... (Mr. Peterson still looks annoyed, but he's beginning to listen.)

Good for you, Sandra! You're hanging in there with a very irritable cardiac patient. It's normal to be thinking to yourself, "Boy, he's so touchy, it's no wonder he has a heart condition!" An inexperienced PT might have become flustered or even left the room. Assertiveness tends to come with age (which is probably why so many elderly patients are cantankerous and demanding), but even a soft-spoken, somewhat shy therapist can focus on the purpose of her communication with such a patient. Sandra knows she must tell Mr. Peterson who she is and what her job is no matter what frame of mind he's in. In the face of his rebuff, she managed to address him by name politely but firmly, and gave her name and title again. She made her purpose clear and never gave in to the temptation to betray anger, fear or disgust. This patient is fortunate to have an understanding therapist who recognizes his needs and her own professional responsibility.

If your patient is a child, remember that same ethic. The child needs to know your name and who you are, especially because children may harbor intense fears about pain and death when they are under professional care. You'll need all your "Informer" skills for the pediatric set.

> THERAPIST: Hi, Andrew. My name is Jeannie Decker. I'm your physical therapist. (she smiles at him and extends her hand to him)
>
> ANDREW: Hi. (he shakes hands tentatively)
>
> THERAPIST: I'm going to help you do some fun exercises for a little while. Then you can watch TV back in your room. Did you ever see the physical therapy room in the hospital?
>
> ANDREW: No. Is it far away?
>
> THERAPIST: It's downstairs. We'll ride the elevator together.
>
> ANDREW: What do they do there?
>
> THERAPIST: Well, there are bicycles you can pedal, but they stay in one place like some of the horses on the merry-go-round. And there are parallel bars so you can hold on when you walk in between them. And there are big mats on the floor. They're really good, because you can lie on the floor to do exercises and it's nice and soft on your back.
>
> ANDREW: Do I have to get a shot?
>
> THERAPIST: Nope. I don't give shots. I'm going to teach you some exercises to help you get strong.
>
> ANDREW: Like Superman?
>
> THERAPIST: Well, maybe not *that* strong, but you can think about Superman while you exercise.
>
> ANDREW: We exercise in school and we go outside in the schoolyard, too.
>
> THERAPIST: Maybe some of these new exercises are like the ones you do in school. You ready to go?
>
> ANDREW: And I can watch TV right after?
>
> THERAPIST: Yes, I'll take you right back here. OK, here we go . . .

Children may not be as concerned about your name and title as they are about whether or not you're going to do something unpleasant to them. They often want reassuring information. Jeannie did well as an informer. She told Andrew what he wanted to know, and she told him without condescending in ways he could understand. He might ask her eventually, "What's your name?" When he does, it will indicate his feeling safe with her and is willingness to draw her into his group of special caregivers.

Well-behaved children like Andrew are every therapist's dream. But if a child is boisterous, inattentive or contrary, your best bet (unless you're one of those wonderful people fresh kids somehow respect) is to take his mother or father along for the therapy session. Ask the parent how you can deal with the child during his therapy so it does him the most good and keeps your sanity intact.

Therapists should feel free to refer a patient to another therapist if they feel the frustrations are at the root of less-than-optimal rapport.

And that referral is OK. Harry Royal, director of physical therapy at Loma Linda University Medical Center in Loma Linda, Calif., recommends being honest enough with yourself to realize it's a "no-go" between you and the patient. But, he said, there's no need to blame yourself if the chemistry just wasn't there. The patient's welfare should overrule a therapist's pride.

Royal also said cardiopulmonary patients in physical therapy may challenge your "Informer" skills.

"The first issue right up front is to adjust yourself to all the things the cardiac patient is aware of—his heart rate, pulse, respiration, blood pressure. . . . Read the chart and progress notes, talk to the physicians and nurses about what's going on with the patient," Royal said. "You need a basis of knowledge about the individual. Put all the pieces from your education together in new ways for each patient. If you don't, you're not even being a therapist." [2]

Essentially, letting the patient know who you are and how you plan to help him or her is the first step. Being well-informed is the next, and most likely, being a "Mensch"—the Yiddish word for "a compassionate person, a real human being"—will allow you to climb that stairway to successful practice.

Going Beyond Introductions

"Opening Night"

Once you've introduced yourself, you may find yourself struggling to go from small talk to the beginning therapeutic range of communication. "Opening Night" is an image that can help you. Consider the first performance of a play on Broadway. The play has to be challenging to the audience and the actors have to create characters people will relate to and remember. An "opener" refers to something in a theatrical production or a book that captures the audience's desire to stay with it.

Your patients may need encouragement to go beyond polite greetings, as in the following situation:

> THERAPIST: What are your questions about your physical therapy, Mr. Ellis?
> PATIENT: Well, how long will it take before I can get rid of this brace on my leg?
> THERAPIST: That varies from patient to patient. Some need two months; others need six.
> PATIENT: God! Six months is a long time!
> THERAPIST: It can certainly seem that way. But let's work on this problem together . . .

The therapist could also have begun with: Where do you think is a good place to start? I imagine you're thinking about your therapy . . . What would you like to talk about? Perhaps something is on your mind? From time to time, you'll be confronted with a patient who insists he or she is not thinking of anything in particular or who says, "It's up to you." Ask the physician or nurse about the patient's reaction if you can. The patient may be an extremely quiet, compliant person, or he or she may be troubled but unable or unwilling to explain. Unless a patient refuses therapy altogether, go ahead with the session using as many encouraging statements as you can muster. Perhaps a patient requires more time to trust you or turn to you for help.

Make statements that call for an answer beyond "yes" or "no." This is an important bit of training, because our "fast information" society fosters multiple choice tests (as opposed to essay tests) and other quick methods of finding things out.

One mother was having a terrible time getting her three-year-old to take her naps. Every afternoon, the mother would say, "Are you ready to take your nap, Melissa?" The child always said no.

"But don't you want to get your beauty sleep?"

"No."

"Well, then, don't you want to grow up to be healthy?"

"No."

"Do you want a spanking?"

"No."

The dialogue became tiresome, and the mother's questions rarely had any effect upon the willful Melissa. A psychologist suggested the mother make a statement instead of asking a question that gave the child the opportunity to run the show and drive the mother crazy.

"Tell Melissa it's nap time," the psychologist said. "Then give her her 'way' in the situation. Ask, 'Do you want to take a nap with the door open or closed?' or 'Would you rather have milk and a cookie before or after your nap?. She can't reasonably say no to either question, and at the same time, she realizes she can't compromise her mother's authority."

The same theory can help the therapist avoid those monosyllabic answers. Questions that begin with "Do you," "Do you want to," "Are you," "Can you," "Will you," "Won't you," "Wouldn't you," "Do you have," "Do you ever," and so on are often satisfied (by the patient, that is) with a yes or no. Try instead to let the question lead into a more complex answer, and take your cue from there.

Acknowledging the Patient

"You Are There"

If you happen to walk into a patient's room at the rehab, hospital or her home, and she's in the midst of doing a puzzle, painting a landscape or knitting a scarf, why not comment pleasantly on that? When you acknowledge the patient in any way, a valuable communication occurs.

> THERAPIST: Good afternoon, Mrs. Turnbull. What a marvelous afghan that's going to be when you finish!
> PATIENT: Hello, Clara. Yes, I've really been working up a storm on it.
> THERAPIST: How are those fingers? Looks like you could crochet a blanket that would cover the world.
> PATIENT: Well, see? My fingers are doin' pretty good for crocheting, (she wiggles fingers of one hand at Clara) but when I go to grab a dish out of the cabinet, they poop out on me.
> THERAPIST: Hmmm, let's see what can be done about that . . .

Clara and Mrs. Turnbull have known each other for a short while since Mrs. Turnbull's occupational therapy began. You may be thinking how much easier it is to use this "You Are There" technique of acknowledgment with a familiar person than a new patient. Of course, that's true, but a sharp eye and a genuine interest in a patient result in any number of ways to acknowledge him or her. A therapist may also encounter a patient who is sitting and staring into space.

> THERAPIST: Mr. Whitmore? It's Clara. Time for your occupational therapy.
> PATIENT: (no response except a nod in greeting)
> THERAPIST: I notice you're wearing a new robe. Looks quite nice.
> PATIENT: My daughter gave it to me for Christmas.
> THERAPIST: Blue is a good color for you. Your daughter must have wanted the robe to match your eyes.
> PATIENT: (chuckles a bit) Oh, sure. Or the ocean. She used to kid me about all the smelly fish I used to catch when . . .

That was a tricky start, but Clara managed to revive Mr. Whitmore's good spirits with her observation of a garment she'd never seen him wear before. She noticed he has blue eyes. Somehow, those observations jogged him into what probably ended up as a pleasant therapeutic communication.

The therapist may also acknowledge a patient's new make-up, necklace, hairdo, shoeshine, belt buckle . . . virtually anything that belongs to the patient that could work into an acknowledging, positive remark. A "negative" observation may be possible when it points out some degree of the patient's progress. For example:

> THERAPIST: Well, well, well, Mr. Salerno, what on earth became of that bum knee of yours? You're standing up straighter than I've ever seen!
> PATIENT: Yeah, not bad, huh? Now I can keep up with my wife when we walk in the neighborhood. Bum knees are for bums, right? (they laugh)

Try to keep the acknowledgment one that directly pertains to the patient. However, there will be times when you really have to reach for the "You Are There" goal. In this case, consider the patient's surroundings, or try to find out something about a new patient ahead of time so you have at least a shred of conversation in store.

Observing Subtle Clues

"On the Lookout"

Acknowledgments travel from a fairly superficial level to a deeper therapeutic level with a technique we call "On the Lookout." Rather than focusing on a patient's new blouse or the like, the therapist picks up on a mood or attitude, which is more difficult to perceive. But acknowledging and, in some sense, challenging a patient's attitude may open a conversation that can affect that patient in many ways.

> THERAPIST: I'm picking up some tense "vibes" from you, Jerry.
> PATIENT: Yeah, I'm kinda nervous. My Mom said she'd be here at 3, and it's 4 o'clock.

Here, the therapist and her teen-aged patient have an easy flow of communication. It didn't take too much prodding to get Jerry to reveal the source of his observable tension. An older patient provides a different dialogue, and a therapist might not be so casual in expressing her perception.

> THERAPIST: Miss Clayborn, you seem on edge. You're clenching your fist, and you're looking away.
> PATIENT: No, I'm just fine.
> THERAPIST: You seem very uncomfortable.
> PATIENT: I'll be all right.
> THERAPIST: I notice that you're not in such good spirits today.
> PATIENT: Oh, sometimes it's hard to . . .

Miss Clayborn's therapist found various ways to express the same perception of her patient's edgy behavior. Sometimes it's necessary to use a few different words until the patient responds. For example, Miss Clayborn denied initially that her fist had anything to do with her mood. The therapist persisted in the interest of the patient. The word "uncomfortable" didn't seem to trigger a response, either. Still, the therapist persisted and used the words "good spirits." Perhaps it was the particular phrase and perhaps it was the therapist's third reference that helped Miss Clayborn start to let out some of her tension—or anger or fear.

Keep in mind there are patients who will not ease some tension by talking, and persistence beyond a reasonable point becomes a futile game. Try to read the patient's signals as accurately as possible. You may have to initiate a conversation later on. If a patient seems unable to open up, perhaps you should consult a psychologist or recommend counseling for the patient. This doesn't mean the "On the Lookout" technique doesn't work or that you've failed. Human behavior has yet to be completely understood. Communication, as effective as it can be, is our link to that understanding.

Other "On the Lookout" phrases include: I perceive that you...Maybe you're uneasy about...I see you're wringing your hands...

With experience, you'll be able to recognize a patient's behavior automatically. The following communication technique offers therapeutic responses to "Lookout" phrases.

Delving Beyond Surface Issues

"Deep Sea Diver"

Using the image of the deep sea diver may be the best way to encourage the therapist to get below the surface with a patient who is reticent or troubled. The diver first has to be well-equipped with a wet suit, oxygen source and a face mask before plunging into the water. Second, he or she has to know the weather and tidal conditions, something about the waters into which he or she is planning to dive, and how to avoid dangers related to diving. Third and most important, he or she has to know how and when to ascend and get back on the shore or boat.

It's not terribly remote from what a therapist faces. Your equipment is your education, your application of it and your willingness to "dive." Then you should find out as much as you can about the patient from the chart, the physician and nurse, the patient and his or her family or other significant people in his or her life. Finally, know when to probe and when to back off. Pushing too hard can do harm in the long run. Particularly avoid this if you foresee enough therapy sessions in which to allow the patient to "emerge" at his or her own pace.

Depending upon the patient's and your personalities, a certain type of "pushing" technique called "tough love" may help in extraordinary circumstances, for example, with patients who are substance abusers. Ask a social worker or psychologist about "tough love" if you feel interested, but most of the time, a combination of caring and good communication skills will serve well.

And now for the "dive":

PATIENT: I was in an accident.
THERAPIST: Tell me some of the things you remember about the accident.
PATIENT: I remember it was late at night...

Another "Deep Sea Dive" may begin this way:

THERAPIST: I see you have a bandage on your head. Please describe what happened to you.
PATIENT: I was thrown through the windshield.
THERAPIST: Tell me about the accident.
PATIENT: It's all kind of a blur, you know. But this car ran a red light and slammed right into me. He was really speeding...

"Deep-sea diving" also applies to emotional distress in cases where there was no car accident or similar traumatic injury. A disease process often dredges up problems related to the patient's lifestyle readjustment, his or her occupational deficits, relationships and motivation for self-care.

PATIENT: I hate this damn hospital.
THERAPIST: Tell me your reasons for saying that, Bob.
PATIENT: The food stinks. The guy next to me coughs all the time. Visiting hours are too short. I hate it all.
THERAPIST: Tell me more. What else?
PATIENT: It's too crowded. I feel like I don't have any of my own space where I can be in peace...

The therapist encouraged Bob to tell about his feelings by saying "Tell me," not at all with the same meaning as the popular rhetorical phrase, "Tell me about it." The first "tell me" conveys genuine interest on the part of the therapist. It is a nonjudgmental response and gives the patient the opportunity to air his concerns without contradiction or interruption. Can you recall how good it sometimes feels just to rant and rave for a while about a problem? The problem must first be acknowledged if a solution is to be sought.

Talking about the less-than-elegant conditions of life in a hospital ward affords Bob a certain amount of relief. The therapist's encouraging words help Bob feel free and safe to say some pretty unflattering things he's been stewing about for days. In releasing his gripes, Bob may go further and communicate on a more intimate level. Perhaps, for instance, he's finding it particularly difficult to cope because he's worried about losing his girlfriend, or that his family won't be proud of him, the former high school basketball champ, now that he's disabled. Complaints about the "small stuff" may be shielding the real issues.

The next time you're talking with a friend who says, "If the landlord raises my rent another dollar, I'll jump" you might find yourself saying, "Tell me about it!" the way a person would use the phrase "*I'll say!*" or "Don't I know it!"

But your friend may surprise you and give you more details about his apartment, his rent or his landlord than you wanted to hear.

Pursuing the Issues

"Mush!"

Once your patient has described his or her problem and some feelings about it, you'll want that patient to continue the communication until a therapeutic plateau has been achieved—relief as a result of having shared the struggle or the power to delve more deeply into emotional disturbances and set up goals to help alleviate them.

Can you picture yourself on a dogsled in Alaska? You're traveling across the snowy plain to your warm shelter, and the dogs know exactly what you mean when you yell, "Mush!"

Of course, if you yell "Mush!" to a patient, she'll probably think you're looney. There are much calmer ways of getting her to pursue her thoughts as she reveals them to you.

PATIENT: My dream in life was to be a concert pianist.
THERAPIST: And now?
PATIENT: And just look at me now. I'm too uncoordinated to make a phone call sometimes.
THERAPIST: Talk to me about that.
PATIENT: My muscles just don't want to do what my brain wants them to do. Why did I have to get this disease?
THERAPIST: Go on, Mary Jean.
PATIENT: Everything was fine before this. I never had to struggle to do things. Maybe I should consider being a writer. I've been thinking about it.
THERAPIST: What then?
PATIENT: Then I wouldn't have to worry about whether I'm coordinated or not. I could dictate into a tape recorder and send the tapes to be transcribed by a typing service. I can still talk, thank God.

The simple things this therapist said to Mary Jean led her gently toward accepting her illness and making an attempt to find a productive, satisfying lifestyle in spite of her deficits. Remember to use the "Mush!" technique with good eye contact and an interested tone. Saying "go on" to a patient as you gaze out the window or down the hall won't have a positive effect. Mary Jean needs a therapist who cares about her and shows it. She's revamping her life's dream; help her stay on track.

Showing Acceptance

"A-OK"

Colloquial English has many ways of expressing acceptance of a communication: Astronaut lingo gave us "everything's A-OK." The use of telegraphic or electronic communication devices produced "Roger Wilco," "I copy" and "I read you." Military jargon includes "aye-aye" and "thumbs up."

Health professionals may not sound as colorful, but their "A-OK" technique is easy and does the job.

> PATIENT: When I sit up, my hip feels weird. Out of place, like. But before the operation, I couldn't sit up at all without it hurting.
> THERAPIST: Mmm. I can imagine.
> PATIENT: People don't realize how a simple little thing like sitting up can mean a lot if you suddenly can't do it.
> THERAPIST: I'm with you on that (nodding).
> PATIENT: Life is what you make it, I guess.
> THERAPIST: Yes.
> PATIENT: It's a good thing for me I got through the surgery. That makes me feel that I can get through anything . . .

While the therapist in this conversation sounds a bit detached, he actually laid the foundation for a more involved communication by giving the patient the whole floor. Be careful, however, of using the "A-OK" technique to excess. The previous dialogue could have included other techniques if the patient needed additional encouragement to talk. Letting the patient know you're following what he or she is saying may suffice in some cases and not in others. The therapist must develop an instinct about this when he or she has a cumulative knowledge of the communication options.

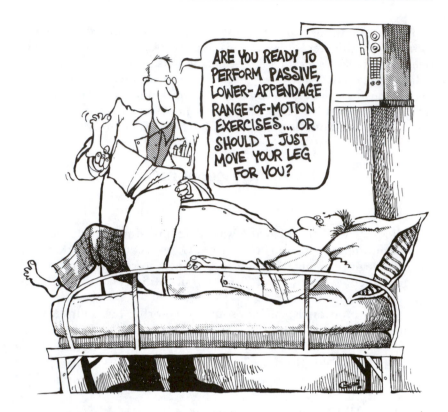

Knowing When to be Quiet

"Silent Treatment"

There's a joke about parents encouraging their very young children to speak and their older children to be quiet. One mother called her son "motor mouth" when he wouldn't stop talking long enough to find out she had a terrible headache.

Then there's the old "Silent Treatment," a punitive method used by spouses or people who find it temporarily distasteful to speak to someone with whom they are angry or disagree.

"Henry and I aren't speaking," one woman confided to her friend. "You can cut the tension around the house with a knife."

While the "Silent Treatment" has a negative reputation, it can be a positive, therapeutic communication technique.

THERAPIST: What were your symptoms before you came to the hospital, Mrs. Crane?

PATIENT: Blackouts. *Total* blackouts. And I got head-aches. (she stops talking) (the therapist remains silent)
PATIENT: Then I was getting confused sometimes.
THERAPIST: Are you still experiencing those symptoms?
PATIENT: Not too much now.
THERAPIST: Maybe you feel a bit more secure here in the hospital. Your cheeks are so nice and rosy.
PATIENT: (laughing) It must be the steroids! I look like a hog!
THERAPIST: (laughing with her) You are really maintaining your sense of humor. That's in your favor. And it gives me the impression you're quite a strong person. What do you think about that?
PATIENT: That's what one of my daughters told me. It's true, I'm pretty strong. But when the doctor first told me I'd have only two years to live if I wanted to forget about the operation, I walked. Two days later I went back and decided to go through with it. They don't know what good the operation will do—at first they were going to use laser beams—but I decided to take a chance.
THERAPIST: I can imagine how difficult that decision was for you. (the patient stops talking and turns her face to the wall) (the therapist also remains silent)
PATIENT: My other daughter hasn't come to see me. Always an excuse—"I have to work," "It's too far..." (the patient's voice breaks and her eyes fill with tears) (the therapist takes her hand without a word; they remain silent, hand-in-hand, for a few moments)
PATIENT: (regaining control of herself) I heard I'll be doing some occupational therapy. It'll be nice to do something useful without the headaches. I couldn't even dress myself sometimes, or make a cup of coffee when I had one of my spells.
THERAPIST: Well, Mrs. Crane, I think you'll be wonderful to work with. Let's both do our best.
PATIENT: (smiling) Now I have something to look forward to!

The complex communication between Mrs. Crane and this compassionate therapist shows that remaining silent at times is not at all representative of a gap or drop in rapport. Mrs. Crane stopped talking whenever she needed to compose her thoughts, and the therapist, who didn't feel the need to fill every pause with sound, gave her the opportunity to do this without interruption.

The therapist also uses other techniques ("You Are There": "rosy cheeks," "you're maintaining your sense of humor"), as you'll find you'll need to do, depending on your patients' responses. Notice how this therapist's "Silent Treatment" blended well with a deliberate gesture: she took the patient's hand. Speech wasn't necessary at that moment, but a connection and an understanding were. The therapist felt unafraid to reach out and her instinct was rewarded. She communicated to Mrs. Crane that she wouldn't "lose" her if it became difficult to speak or if she began to cry. Part of being a therapist is allowing a patient to release his or her feelings in a safe way.

Of course, it's not *always* appropriate to hold a patient's hand. There's probably no concrete criterion for when to do it or not; you just have to read the signals.

Staying with the Patient

"Yours Truly"

In much the same way that holding a patient's hand at the right time provides comfort, so can telling your patient you'll stay with him or her as long as he or she feels you're comforting. This technique may be especially useful with cardiac or pulmonary patients in physical therapy. These patients need to relax as much as possible and to be reassured you'll be there if they feel distressed. Chest pain or severe coughing can be traumatic, which adds to these patients' sense of fear.

> PATIENT: I'm in lousy shape. When I cough, I get short of breath—the way you feel after you ran the 40-yard dash. (starts to breathe laboriously and cough) (the therapist stays with him and says nothing) (patient settles down again)
> THERAPIST: How do you feel now?
> PATIENT: Like I'm gonna start coughing all over the place again.
> THERAPIST: I'll sit with you. You try to relax a bit before we continue your therapy.
> PATIENT: OK. Thanks. That's good.

The "Yours Truly" phrases, such as "I'll stay with you," "I'm here," "I'm with you now" or "I'll sit with you" appeal to the human need for emotional support. They may not seem like therapy or a major method of communication because we often say them instinctively when we're not in the therapist-patient setting. How many times have you heard a mother say to her child, "Mommy's here with you. I'll always be with you" when the child feels afraid or ill? Why do you think a child calls out to his or her parents in the first place? Because he or she seeks the comfort they consistently offer.

Did you ever think about why teen-aged girls go to the ladies' room in pairs or groups? Most likely they're more secure and less self-conscious in a group than they are when they have to get up and walk across a room alone. It may sound silly, but it grows into a larger concept of "moral support." Almost everyone has asked someone to "just be there" during a crucial moment.

In the therapist-patient relationship, however, use the "Yours Truly" communication with discrimination. Recognize when a patient has accepted a "sick role," which means he or she is resigned to living the life of an invalid and has become overly dependent on his or her family and caregivers. "Sick role" patients often become demanding and impossible to deal with when they expect everyone to jump at their tiniest whims. As a therapist, you have to decide just how long to stay with a patient and whether or not the support is warranted and therapeutic. Don't stay with a patient out of a sense of guilt or pity. Patients don't need pity. They need help to strengthen or regain their physical and occupational functions.

Quick Guide to Techniques

1. THE INFORMER—"I'm Sally Jones, physical therapist . . ."
2. OPENING NIGHT—"What are your feelings about . . . ?"
3. YOU ARE THERE—"How nice your hair looks today . . ."
4. ON THE LOOKOUT—"I notice you're trembling . . ."
5. DEEP SEA DIVER—"Tell me more . . ."
6. MUSH!—"Go on . . ."
7. A-OK—"Yes, I follow . . ."
8. SILENT TREATMENT—(wait and observe)
9. YOURS TRULY—"I'll stay with you . . ."
10. SAY WHAT?—"Please explain . . ."
11. WHICH CAME FIRST?—"What happened after that . . . ?"
12. COMPARISON SHOPPING—"Was it something like . . . ?"
13. PLAY IT AGAIN, SAM—"Run that by me once more . . ."
14. RETURN TO SENDER—"Return to Sender?"

15. ZOOM LENS—"Let's focus on that . . ."
16. POW-WOW—"Let's make sure we're on the same wave length . . ."
17. JUST THE FACTS, MA'AM—"I don't hear any voices . . ."
18. DOUBTING THOMAS—"That's hard to believe . . ."
19. THE TRANSLATOR—"So you're suggesting . . . ?"
20. WHAT'S IT WORTH?—"How does that make a difference . . . ?"
21. A LITTLE HINT—"You feel misunderstood . . . ?"
22. WHAT A TEAM!—"Maybe together we can solve this . . ."
23. IN A NUTSHELL—"So far we talked about . . ."
24. LIGHTS! CAMERA! ACTION!—"How are you going to handle . . . ?"

Hold Off on Nontherapeutic Communication

1. "You're going to be fine . . ."
2. "Don't say things like that . . ."
3. "I don't want to hear it . . ."
4. "You're wrong . . ."
5. "You're absolutely right . . ."
6. "You ought to . . .
7. "So if you're numb, how come you're still talking?"
8. "Do you know where you are?"
9. "Still think you're an ace linebacker?"
10. "That's ridiculous, no one here could have done that . . ."
11. "Why . . . ?"
12. "Oh, you're not the only one who feels that way . . ."
13. "Looks like rain . . ."
14. "What you really mean is . . ."
15. "What a worry-wart!"
16. "You're imagination is running away with you . . ."
17. "It's your own fault . . ."
18. "Prove it . . ."
19. "You'd better do it now or you'll never do it . . ."
20. "Nurse Baker? Yeah, she's awful . . ."

Clarifying the Patient's Meaning

"Say What?"

"... And then we'll catch a few birds in the moon-June-spoon and see what the boys are throwing down before we book."

Give up?

The translation is: "We'll pick up a few girls before nighttime and listen to the band before we leave." Of course, these phrases are outdated by at least 20 years, but they illuminate the reason a therapist should ask patients to rephrase their statements when they are not understood. What could be worse than having no idea what a patient has said?

While patients may not use words you cannot define or sentence structures you do not recognize, they *can* say things you'll want them to clarify.

> PATIENT: If I can't go home soon, things are gonna explode around here.
> THERAPIST: I'm not sure I understand what you mean, Sam.
> PATIENT: You know, I'm goin' nuts in this freakin' place.
> THERAPIST: Would you explain that further? I'm concerned about you. Let's hear it.

It's not easy to deal sympathetically with a patient who seems to be throwing all your good efforts for his welfare back in your face. Asking him to explain his feelings offers him an opportunity to vent his feeling of being trapped by his physical disability. Sam knows this therapist really is interested in him. Notice that the therapist asked Sam if he would explain but did not wait for Sam to brush him off. Instead, the therapist expressed a genuine concern followed by a gentle imperative.

What a difference in this version:

> PATIENT: If I can't go home soon, things are gonna explode around here.
> THERAPIST: So what are you, an explosives expert?
> PATIENT: What do you know? I'd like to put a stick of dynamite ...

Well, let's not continue this shameful excuse for a conversation. In it the therapist completely ignored the patient's sense of desperation.

He attacked the patient in a sarcastic, confrontational tone and deserved the nasty response. Nothing was accomplished and ill-feelings resulted.

Much more advisable is giving a patient the opportunity to detail his emotions. Use phrases such as, "Go over that again," "I don't follow—tell me that again" or "Could you explain more about that to me?"

Also, listen carefully to the explanation. If you don't understand even after the patient tries to clarify, it may not be therapeutic to repeat the same phrase you used three minutes before. The patient might become annoyed that he cannot make himself understood. Put yourself in the patient's shoes: Would you appreciate being asked over and over to explain one sentence?

Find another approach to get a clearer picture. The patient may benefit from getting a clearer picture for himself. Asking him, "What do you mean?" or "What are you saying?" often triggers his own ability to reach the real purpose of the communication.

Establishing Chronological Order

"Which Came First?"

Sometimes a patient clouds what she's trying to say because she's not putting events in the right order. Keeping in mind the old question, "Which came first, the chicken or the egg?" helps your patients sort out what's happened to them or who said what to them and when.

> PATIENT: I can't get on a bus without feeling like I'm going to throw up. My friend Alison always rides the bus with me.
> THERAPIST: Karen, did you have those feelings of nausea before or after you started your medication?
> PATIENT: After, I guess. I'm not sure.
> THERAPIST: And did Alison ride with you when you were taking the medication?
> PATIENT: We were little kids when we took the bus to school together and once I threw up and Alison went to the bus driver for help.
> THERAPIST: Oh, I see. So you started the medicine a month ago, and when you take a bus you feel nauseated.
> PATIENT: Yes. It's terrible. I can't go anywhere.
> THERAPIST: And it reminds you of the time you threw up on the schoolbus?

PATIENT: Yes. That must've been 20 years ago.
THERAPIST: And you remember how Alison got help for you when that happened?
PATIENT: She did. She was my best friend.
THERAPIST: OK. Let me make sure I understand. You're feeling nauseated as a side effect of your pills, and the feeling gets worse when you're on the bus, right?
PATIENT: Yes.
THERAPIST: But Alison is part of your past, is that right, too?
PATIENT: Right.
THERAPIST: She doesn't still ride the bus with you?
PATIENT: No, that was a long time ago. I still think about her though.
THERAPIST: She gave you some moral support when you felt sick.
PATIENT: Exactly.
THERAPIST: Karen, when was the last time you took a bus?
PATIENT: This morning on my way here . . .

Because this dialogue could go on, let's end it at this point and recap the situation on a deeper level. The therapist determined that Karen's reaction to the drugs dredged up her fear of losing control of herself (as she did when she was a child) and not having Alison around to comfort her.

At first, Karen told the therapist she feels nauseated on buses, so she rides with her friend Alison. Karen needed to separate the current event, the side effect of her medicine, from a childhood memory. She also needed to confront the patient's feelings of isolation. Perhaps she was seeking in her therapist the moral support Alison once supplied. A PT or OT who suspects a patient has emotional problems that may interfere with therapy sessions should consult a social worker or psychologist for possible referral.

Many patients you will encounter for physical or occupational therapy will be essentially free of emotional disturbances and your conversations will be less probing than the one with Karen. Whenever a patient gives you information about his or her condition that requires your services, however, he or she may need help putting events in order. You can ask directly, "Which came first?" or "When did you first notice symptoms?"

Other phrases you can use include: "What happened before that?"

"What was going on at the time?" "And after that?" "Tell me what led up to your condition now."

If your patient does not remember, consult his or her chart. Both you and your patient will function better if there is a sense of order.

Verbalizing Physical Sensations

"Comparison Shopping"

We are a society of shoppers. We adore getting the best bargain, too, and some people go from store to store pricing that same sweater or appliance or sofa until they've found what they think is the lowest price. Often, a shopper triumphs by discovering a similar item that's a different brand at a lower price.

In terms of communicative therapy, asking a patient to compare an experience to something else can result in the therapist's having a much sharper idea of how the patient feels and perhaps what to do about it.

> THERAPIST: Ava, give me a better picture of what's going on with you. What's your pain like?
> PATIENT: It's like being stretched suddenly and my muscles feel real tight.
> THERAPIST: Is that something you could call a spasm?
> PATIENT: Yeah, I think so.
> THERAPIST: Have you ever felt something like that before in the other leg?

People can often describe pain by comparing it to a dull throb, a knife, a needle, a vise or crushed feeling. Allow your patient to give her own description if she can even if you're tempted to put words such as "squeezing" or "sharp" in her mouth. A fundamental tenet of dealing with a patient's pain holds that pain is whatever the patient says it is. Consider the implication of this dialogue:

> PATIENT: Henry, this ankle feels as though a big fish with sharp teeth is biting me in the water.
> THERAPIST: That can't be, Sarah. You had your pain medication only 45 minutes before you came down to PT.

Where does that response leave Sarah? Henry discounted her pain, which she described as intense, if you can imagine what being bitten on a delicate ankle would feel like. Furthermore, Sarah would justifiably feel insulted by Henry's short-sighted words. How dare he call her a liar when she's in such distress! Perhaps he doesn't realize the possibility that Sarah's tolerance for the pain medication has increased and the dose she was given no longer works against her pain. As Sarah soaks her ankle in the whirlpool, she might become so angry with Henry for not taking her seriously that she decides, "I'll never try to tell HIM anything ever again! He just doesn't understand."

Why let that happen? Think of how you'd feel if you said to one of your caregivers, "I can't breathe" and she said, "Don't be silly. You're breathing or you couldn't talk." Could you blame a patient for complaining to someone else in search of relief? Recharge your sensitivities by turning the tables for a moment. Recognize what severe pain does to a person—it robs him or her of the pleasure of living. It sounds drastic because it is.

And you can't argue pain. Unless you're experiencing it first hand, stop yourself from saying to your patient, "There, now, try to relax. It's all right" or "Oh, come on now, it's not that bad." It certainly is NOT all right, so don't feed your patient any superficial denial. And listen to that other omniscient tone: "It's not that bad." The therapist who says that must feel very self-important to think he or she can neatly shelve someone's trauma.

If Lu Ann tells you she feels as though a mule is sitting on her back, consider her description carefully and assess not whether she feels this or not, but what could be causing that type of pain.

Also consider the patient who smiles or even laughs and jokes when describing pain.

> THERAPIST: What's the pain like now, Jack?
> PATIENT: It's like the guy who's so religious he got canonized—with a real cannon.

You may not hear anything like that very often, but if you do, it would be appropriate to laugh with the patient while doing everything you can to help him. People use humor as a defense mechanism against stressful or painful situations. Jack mustered up a clever line through an episode of shortness of breath and chest pain. A sharp therapist heard Jack express a devastating physical experience despite his humor. It's also possible that Jack is like the TV character Hawkeye Pierce, who could crack jokes during a visit from the ghost of Christmas Future.

Whatever the patient's profile, take his or her pain as seriously as the patient does. In the case of a known hypochondriac who insists on wailing long and loudly over a hangnail, test your therapeutic communication skills. This type of patient probably needs to vent his or her troubles in more specific ways and be encouraged to re-evaluate them in a more realistic manner. Yelling "Pain!" has long been an attention-getter—most of the time for understandable reasons.

When pain is not the issue, a patient may describe a dizzy spell, a lack of strength, or coordination or other deficit as "a floating feeling" or "like trying to run in a dream when your legs feel heavy."

The "Comparison Shopping" technique works to allow a patient to air his or her problem and gives the therapist at least a dual level of insight.

Restating the Patient's Description

"Play It Again, Sam"

Once your patient has verbalized what she is experiencing, you may want to restate her words to confirm to her that you're concerned and listening carefully to her. We call this technique "Play It Again, Sam" because in the movie, "Casablanca," the two romantic leads, played by Humphrey Bogart and Ingrid Bergman, wanted to hear the song "As Time Goes By" because it brought back memories for them.

Bring back your patient's words or general ideas, then, to recapture the mood and perhaps call forth subconscious levels of the patient's communication.

> PATIENT: I keep thinking I'm at the ballet *barre* doing stretches and *pliés*. I think about it all the time.
> THERAPIST: You're worried about missing your dance classes.
> PATIENT: I guess so. No matter what happens, I want to be a dancer.
> THERAPIST: Dancing is an important part of your life.

The dancer, temporarily disabled and disconnected from an aesthetic, fulfilling aspect of herself and her world, has maintained her vision. The therapist in this instance underscored and broadened what she expressed.

A therapist could miss a patient's point, however, to a sad result.

> PATIENT: I think about dancing all the time. I can't get it out of my mind.
> THERAPIST: Well, now, you shouldn't be thinking about

> dancing in your condition. There are other activities you
> should try, like needlepoint . . .

Oh, woe! He dashed his patient's communication and substituted a discount, at best, and an insult, at worst. This aspiring performer would turn off to such remarks. She subtly reached out for emotional support, but the unfortunate therapist didn't realize her situation beyond her words. He wasn't really listening well or reading her body language. He paid no attention to the enthusiastic tone and pace of her voice; he never heard of "Deep Sea Diving" to encourage a patient to express deep-seated feelings.

His rendition of "Play It Again, Sam" does not jibe at all with therapeutic communication. An assertive patient might have responded, "You've discounted what I was saying, Charles, and I feel uncomfortable because of that. I wanted to share something that's important to me, and you brushed it off."

Charles might then have straightened out the situation and made therapeutic amends. "I'm so sorry, Deborah. You're right. I was preoccupied when you began to talk. I was thinking about Larry's surgery this morning. Let's make sure we talk about your dancing during our session tomorrow. I remember how excited I always was to talk about my career, and your dancing must really be wonderful. What do you say?"

Deborah agreed and the professional relationship survived. Charles admitted his mistake, apologized and offered the patient a "makeup" time. He stretched back into his own psyche to the days when he thought incessantly about becoming a therapist and shared that with her.

But don't expect patients to be as forgiving and enlightening as Deborah was to Charles. Most patients would choke down feelings of resentment, not realizing they don't need anyone's permission to say what's really on their minds. It's up to the therapist to hone his perception and use his therapeutic communication techniques toward the patient's physical and mental well-being.

Reflective Listening

"Return To Sender"

The lyrics of an old Elvis Presley song, "Return to sender, address unknown . . . ," tell a story of a young man who pours his heart out to the girl of his dreams in a letter, but he's lost her forever. His letter comes back unopened. He has no chance of communicating with her.

For the therapist, "Return to Sender" means giving a patient's own words back to him or her in such a way that he or she will continue to talk until the expression is gratifying.

> PATIENT: I'm dead from the waist down.
> THERAPIST: You're dead from the waist down?
> PATIENT: Yeah. I feel like half a person. I can talk and move my arms, but that's only half of what everybody else can do . . .

In this dialogue, all the therapist had to do was repeat the patient's words to him as a question. The patient was willing to explain using different words and a more direct image. By mirroring the patient's statement, the therapist communicated her interest in the deeper meanings of what the patient said.

Another version of "Return to Sender" involves a patient asking for direction:

> PATIENT: Carol, do you think going home will mean a setback?
> THERAPIST: Do *you* think going home will mean a setback?

In most cases, common sense tells us to let the patient's viewpoints take center stage. Carol achieved that through the "Return to Sender" technique above, and at the same time, she gently prodded the patient to think harder about her situation. If Carol had been less compassionate and perceptive, she might have given a fast, "Nah, probably not—chin up" response that might have left the patient stewing unnecessarily and feeling short-changed.

It also might have short-changed the therapist of the opportunity to give crucial caring at a crucial time.

Focusing on Patient Concerns

"Zoom Lens"

A zoom lens is a special lens for a camera that helps the photographer take a close-up picture of someone from quite a distance. Very often, the subject does not know he's being photographed. The zoom lens magnifies the selected subject so it becomes the largest or main part of the composition.

A verbal "zoom lens" fills the "picture" with one of the patient's significant statements.

> PATIENT: I can't wait to be steady enough to put on some mascara. Ever since I came here I've been more concerned with being able to feed myself than anything else.
> THERAPIST: You seem to be progressing nicely. I enjoy being able to help you get back into your daily activities.
> PATIENT: I suppose it's time to look like a woman again.
> THERAPIST: Hmm . . . Let's focus on that point. It sounds like an important step for you . . .

The OT here understood exactly what her patient communicated: She's progressed to the point of recognizing a need beyond basic ADL skills. She wants to enhance her femininity. The therapist knew her patient's history as an attractive young woman. Her desire to apply makeup as she once had as a part of her normal routine signaled her increasing desire to function independently and purposefully in society.

Phrases such as "Let's stay with that point," "That's worth a closer look" or "it seems you've reached an important point here" encourage a patient to explore one thing thoroughly before going on to something else. They also convey that the therapist is more interested in the patient than in quitting time.

Just as a zoom lens can create a dramatic picture, a therapist with the appropriate words can enlarge his or her patient's major concerns—the better to see them and take care of them.

Understanding Each Other

"Pow-Wow"

When a strategy had to be worked out in the American Indian community, the men got together, smoked a peace-pipe and discussed the issue until they felt confident they knew what to do. They called such a meeting a "pow-wow," which has become a commonly used term in nearly every American community.

A pow-wow with a patient also refers to coming to a mutual understanding. Among the phrases a therapist can use are: "When you use the word "tired," do you mean physically or emotionally?" "My understanding of what you said is . . . Does that agree with yours?" "I want to make sure we're both on the same wave length when it comes to . . ." "Are we talking about the same time period?" "Let's recap and

see if our understanding of the situation works the same way..."
"Did you mean to bring up the subject of...?" "Tell me if what I'm
hearing is what you're really saying..." "Do we agree on...?"

Each therapist has to find his or her own way of making sure that
therapist and patient stay on the mark with each other so significant
communication does not get lost in the shuffle. Remember the "Pow-
wow." It's an accessible image for a therapeutic technique professionals often overlook.

Maintaining a Reality Base

"Just The Facts, Ma'am"

Remember the television detective series "Dragnet"? The weary but
astute detective would often have to prompt a woman who gave a lot
of extraneous opinions with, "Just the facts, ma'am."

The series was so popular that "Just the facts, ma'am" became part
of the American vocabulary. A confused patient, or a patient who is
dodging the truth for whatever reason, may start going 'round and
'round an issue instead of dealing directly and factually with it.

PTs and OTs can encounter patients with mental disorders. It's
probably true that we're all somewhat neurotic and we try to laugh
through it. But what has come to be called "functional neurosis" does
not pose the same communication problems as more serious mental
illness does.

> PATIENT: You're Mary, aren't you?
> THERAPIST: Yes, my name is Mary...
> PATIENT: Jesus told me you'd come.
> THERAPIST: Mrs. Guglio, I'm Mary Smith, your physical
> therapist. I'm not the "Mary" you'd like to think.
> PATIENT: Oh, no, you're the one. That man by the win-
> dow told me for sure.
> THERAPIST: I see no one else in this room. No one is at
> the window.
> PATIENT: Then who are you?
> THERAPIST: My name is Mary Smith, Mrs. Guglio. I'm a
> physical therapist here at the hospital...

When a therapist is not informed that Mrs. Guglio is schizophrenic
in addition to being a below-the-knee amputee who needs physical
therapy, she may feel startled by an encounter like the one above.
Mary Smith handled it well. She identified herself, and she presented
Mrs. Guglio with "Just the Facts." Mary's response to the patient's

expecting the Virgin Mary was a realistic one. (When Mary told this story to some other members of the health care team, she said, "It would have been a lot easier if my name had been Arlene or Debbie!")

When Mrs. Guglio spoke of "that man by the window," Mary gave her a response rooted in reality: I don't see anyone else here. Some caregivers feel they should humor a patient, but consider the nontherapeutic aspect of saying: "Oh, yes. That man tells a lot of people strange things, doesn't he?"

Reinforcing an unrealistic communication shows no real respect for the patient. If a mentally ill patient makes you nervous, practice all the reality-oriented communication you can. Don't be afraid to cross the patient's "view." Your job is to help him or her fight the illness, not fester in it.

While maintaining reality, however, avoid saying, "You must be crazy" or "When was the last time you saw your psychiatrist?" Do discuss the patient with other professionals who deal with him or her to find out what the best—and team—approach is to be taken.

PTs and OTs may also deal with veterans suffering from post-traumatic stress disorder. One Vietnam veteran, now in his forties, had a difficult time during an occupational therapy session. He and the therapist, Patricia, sat at the table near a large window in the activities room. They spoke quietly and the patient performed some coordination exercises.

Suddenly, the sky turned dark gray and rain accompanied a loud clap of thunder. The patient screamed and threw his body behind a nearby couch. The situation worsened when the thunder sounded again, this time with lightning. Conditioned by the terrors of his war experiences, the patient covered his head with his arms and trembled.

Patricia went to him and put a hand on his shoulder.

"Gary, it's Patricia. I'll stay with you until the thunder stops."

Gary accepted her offer but said nothing for a while.

Eventually, he got up and composed himself. When Patricia suggested they resume the therapy, he agreed. Her technique "Just the Facts" combined well with "Yours Truly." She offered her time and understanding while letting him know the noise was thunder, not shellfire.

Expressing Healthy Skepticism

"Doubting Thomas"

According to John 20: 24-29, the apostle Thomas doubted Jesus' resurrection until he had proof of it. Someone who doubts habitually might be called a "doubting Thomas."

Voicing doubt in response to a patient who communicates a delusion or otherwise unrealistic image shows the patient you want to acknowledge and consider what he says. It also lets the patient know he can rethink what he's saying without being rejected or judged.

>   PATIENT: I did 90 sit-ups last night.
>   THERAPIST: That's difficult to believe!

To a patient known to the caregiver as unable to do that vigorous an exercise, the therapist might also have said, "Really?" or "Isn't that unusual?"

However, if he tells you he has shooting pains in his hand, but you see he's had that arm amputated, avoid saying, "That sounds weird to me!" He may be describing phantom pain and not a psychotic episode.

Also, you don't want to start an argument with your patient. It would be ludicrous to say to the patient's report of having done 90 sit-ups, "You did not!" Instead, try to use another communication technique that could give the patient an opportunity to explore an underlying feeling or meaning of his statement. For example, you might say, "You did 90 sit-ups?" or "It sounds as though you're suggesting you're feeling stronger lately." Then let the patient re-evaluate his words.

When you use the "Doubting Thomas" technique, remember to stay within a nonthreatening framework.

Translating

"The Translator"

At times, a patient will make a startling statement that doesn't precisely communicate his feelings. The therapist's task here is to "translate" so a patient becomes able to connect with what he's saying on a deeper level.

>   PATIENT: I'm on Mars.
>   THERAPIST: Are you thinking you're feeling alienated from everything?

This therapist "translated" well. He listened to the patient's words without reacting in a negative, confrontational way. Another version of "The Translator" also involves listening carefully to a patient's tone and observing his body language and facial expression.

PATIENT: I'm dead.

THERAPIST: Carla, is it that you feel life seems meaningless to you?

Here, the translation can become a stock response. Depressed and angry about an illness or injury, many patients have said this and similar things referring to death, numbness or nothingness. How rejecting it would be for a therapist to say, "Don't be a fool." Again, there can't be too much emphasis on allowing a patient to release his or her feelings toward the goal of pursuing optimal well-being.

Assessing Progress

"What's It Worth"

As your patients progress, encourage them to survey their feelings and decide how they can continue with or change their situations. Just as you review their charts regularly, assess their physical and emotional states and determine their needs accordingly, so too can they participate in the evaluation process.

"What's It Worth?" That's the question you ask yourself when you're contemplating spending a large sum of money on a house or car, or when you're trying to figure out how you're going to spend a great deal of time. You weigh the item or situation in your mind to determine its worth to you.

Try a "What's It Worth?" technique with a patient in these ways: Let's go over your progress notes and see what else you have to do... How do you feel about your experiences...? How has this experience changed your thinking...? What contributes to your progress...? What factors seem to undermine your progress...? What seems to add to your pain...? How have others helped you...? How have others hindered you...? What are your emotional needs...? What are you physical needs...? How are you perceiving your present activities...?

Each of these openers is designed to help a patient come to some conclusions about his or her life. A disabled patient must make many temporary or permanent adjustments, which in a host of cases means frustration, pain and other difficulties. When a realistic, thorough assessment can be made, a patient has a better chance of taking significant steps forward.

Tuning Your Third Ear

"A Little Hint"

When Donna was a child, she would often drop hints about what present she would like her parents to get for her birthday.

As an adult and professional therapist, Donna hears "hints" patients give when discussing their feelings. The therapist's ear should be trained to hear these little hints and help patients verbalize them in broader terms.

> PATIENT: Going through all these games is stupid. I've had it with this "Busy Box" thing.
> THERAPIST: Maybe your rehabilitation adjustments remind you of some childhood frustrations?

The OT heard her patient's anger through the attack of the exercise, addressed it promptly and opened a safe line of communication for her patient. She took the "hint"—few hints from patients are subtle.

> PATIENT: If I have to go through life in this wheelchair, I might as well be dead. I'm no man like this. Women want real men.
> THERAPIST: You feel your sexuality has been challenged?
> PATIENT: Well, how would *you* feel if you thought nobody would even look twice at you—if they knew you were paralyzed from the waist down?
> THERAPIST: I hear your fear of sexual rejection. Explain more about that to me.
> PATIENT: I'm a fun-loving guy. I used to, well, you know, do it a lot. I liked thinking I was a real man.
> THERAPIST: Sex gave you a great deal of pleasure.
> PATIENT: Yeah—c'mon, everybody likes it. But who'd want me now? I can't . . . my body is different now.
> THERAPIST: You feel you'd have trouble going back to sexual relations?
> PATIENT: I can *think* about sex, but I don't know what it'll be like to actually try it again. How could I get a girl to want to be with me?
> THERAPIST: Is it that you feel undesirable to women?
> PATIENT: I'm not bad-looking, but women would probably think I'd be better as a friend than as a lover. You know what I mean. Why should they get involved with Mr. Instant Problems? They want a guy to take care of *them*.
> THERAPIST: It sounds as though you believe women only want one thing from a man! (patient chuckles)
> PATIENT: OK, I get what you're saying. I was brought up old-fashioned. Women's lib never did much for me . . .

The therapist maintained her professional demeanor even during a fairly emotional communication on an intimate subject. She translated the patient's words into direct overviews ("You feel your sexuality has been challenged?"). She didn't act embarrassed and she didn't reprimand or belittle the patient's concerns. She allowed him time to vent, and she even got him to laugh a bit, which broke his tension and helped him see that at that point he was being narrow-minded.

The exchange was moving in a therapeutic direction. Perhaps the therapist referred the patient to a counselor who could help him cope with sexual readjustment. An OT or PT cannot play the role of a psychologist, but a patient may begin to open up with a sympathetic caregiver. Referral should be recognized as a professional responsibility. If communication between you and a patient "runs away" emotionally, tell your patient you believe he would benefit from taking his problem to a specially trained professional. And explain that you want him to have the best possible care.

Emphasizing Teamwork

"What A Team!"

The sports world has its stars, the Hall-of-Famers whose names have become synonymous with pride and admiration and inspiration. But where would the sports world be without its teams? Imagine even the most marvelous player out in the field by himself or herself. Imagine empty bleachers and stadiums without all the cheers and shouts of "Go, team, go!"

Now imagine a patient—even the most independent patient with the brightest of futures—left to rehabilitate himself or herself without an expert's plan for his or her care and without encouraging words. In the absence of the health care team, people might take longer to recover or recover only to endure deficits no one taught them to work against. Recovery does not always go hand-in-hand with rehabilitation.

As a therapist, you can offer your patients a team effort toward rehabilitation by using the following phrases: Perhaps together we can solve the problem of . . . Let's figure out how you can . . . We can work together to . . . How about you and I talking about . . . Let's both decide on a plan for . . . The two of us can discover . . . We'll create a plan so that . . . If we collaborate on this, we can . . .

Few words of comfort have as much impact on a patient who's been through a grueling time as "let's," "together" and "we." Every patient needs support in one way or another. For some, support

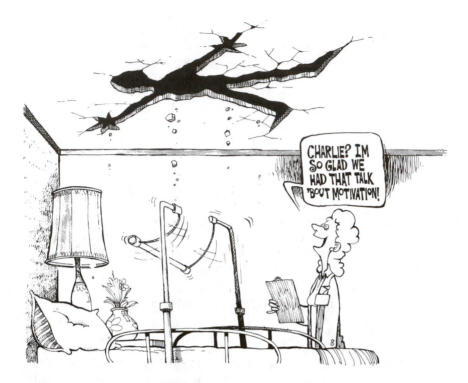

means a little caring conversation; for others, it may involve extensive planning and unflagging encouragement.

The success of the team, however, depends upon each player's giving it all his or her effort. Make it clear to your patients that they are key "players." They have to be willing to meet you at least half-way if the team is going to exist at all.

When your "team" wins, remember to pat each other on the back. Tell a patient he or she did a fine job. Say that his or her courage was a real example. And be prepared to accept a few compliments on your work from the patient.

For those who have a difficult time accepting a compliment graciously, stock a few possible responses so you don't end up tongue-tied and blurting out: "Oh, I didn't really do anything" or "That's just part of my job."

Think of how rejected you would feel if you complimented someone sincerely and it was tossed aside. What a downer! But it's not uncommon for people to respond negatively to praise or gratitude no matter how much they actually appreciate it. It's just that they are caught off guard and feel embarrassed to show their pleasure. We're taught to be modest, but it's easier for you and the patient to share your true feelings.

> PATIENT: I don't know what I would have done without you. You were great.
> THERAPIST: Thanks so much, Peter. Whenever I'm feeling low, I'll remember what you said today.

The therapist could also have said, "That means a lot to me" or "When you say that, I feel very happy." Whatever words seem natural to you, see that they are accepting words, warm, simple and appropriate.

Summarizing What the Patient Says

"In a Nutshell"

"Boy meets girl. Girl loves another. Boy fights for her, defeats the opponent. Girl marries boy. They live happily ever after."

It may sound corny, but it's a fair summary of many books, plays and movies. It tells the whole story in a nutshell.

At times, you'll find it necessary to put your patient's story in a nutshell. A summary—the bare bones of the situation—helps clarify and sort out primary information for you and the patient. Summarizing what a patient has said to you lets him or her know you're not only listening, but you're working toward a real understanding. Also, you're giving the patient a chance to set the record straight if there is a misunderstanding.

Some phrases you can use are: Up to now, you've said ... So far we've talked about ... Since you began your therapy, you've ... Let me see if I have the whole picture ... This is what we've been discussing ... Let's go over the situation ... Here's what I understand to this point ... These seem to be the facts as of now ... Have I missed anything so far?

Frequent "nutshell" discussion may be a significant way for you to keep abreast of your patient's physical and emotional condition. You can become overwhelmed by details and lose sight of the basics as data on your patient accumulate. A little nutshell keeps you focused on long-term goals for your patient—such as "living happily ever after."

Offering Guidance

"Lights! Camera! Action!"

A therapist has to be a good director when a patient experiences problems, but a director doesn't necessarily tell an actor what to do. Instead, he or she guides the actor's ideas and instincts into action. The same can be accomplished with patients.

> PATIENT: It makes me so mad when she treats me like a baby.
> THERAPIST: How are you going to handle anger in a positive way, John?

Ask a patient what course of action he's going to take. Asking reinforces that he is in control of himself and can participate in his care plan.

> PATIENT: Whenever I'm supposed to have a therapy session, I get really nervous and think I'll fail.
> THERAPIST: What do you think you can do the next time you feel that way?

You may be surprised at how well a patient can map out a method that's effective. If a patient seems lost in the situation, find other therapeutic communication techniques to help him verbalize the problem and eventually reach a conclusion. Before action can be taken, he has to see his situation realistically, and he has to develop his strengths. Physical and occupational therapists should provide support as a patient struggles to answer some important questions for himself.

Interpreting Body Language

"Your Body Speaks"

Did you ever notice how some people stick out their tongues or have a funny scowl on their faces when they're concentrating?

Have you ever gone into someone's office and found yourself having a serious discussion with the soles of his shoes?

Can you remember trying to settle a point with a girlfriend who folded her arms or turned her head away from you?

Ever watch a child hang her head or move nervously as a teacher reprimands her?

These are examples of body language—mannerisms and expressions made by your body from head to toe without words.

A therapist who gives a patient her full attention, faces him, sits with a relaxed posture, adopts an appropriate facial expression, has a smooth pace and pitch to her voice, and maintains good eye contact exhibits open or welcoming body language.

Imagine how you would feel if you were the patient and the therapist was reading, cracking her knuckles or filing her nails as you spoke. You would be left standing alone, talking to yourself. And chances are you would hate that, because it's closed—and off-putting—body language.

There are infinite varieties of behavior that indicate anxiety, nervousness and discomfort. A therapist should become attuned to any behavior that seems excessive or particularly expressive. Examples are:

hand-wringing
fist-clenching
teeth-clenching
lip-biting
wincing eyes
looking up or down eyes closed or staring
hair-twirling
fidgeting with clothing, jewelry or other object
leg- or foot-shaking
finger-tapping
picking at crumbs, lint, linens or part of the body
blushing/flushing
becoming livid ("white-as-a-ghost")
falling asleep
knitting the brow
hand covering mouth, eyes, face, ears
hand on chest or throat
arms folded
hands in pockets
head turned away up or down
body turned away
legs crossed at knees or ankles
sitting at the edge of a chair
trembling
eyes watering or filling
hyperventilating or other irregular breathing
rubbing

shrugging or other turning or lifting of shoulders
gum-chewing or cracking
obscene gestures
gestures indicating "stop," "go," and so on, such as putting finger
   to lips, meaning "sh!"
smiling (appropriately or inappropriately)
raising the eyebrows

The list goes on, and as you observe your patients, you will begin to recognize and address a point not verbalized. Try to determine which bodily behaviors are significant, however. A woman who adjusts her eyeglasses or a man who scratches his head momentarily may not be exhibiting any emotions.

And you should not feel you cannot make a move lest your patient "read" you incorrectly. Just be aware of behavior that might be an obvious betrayal of feelings when a situation may provoke it. If a patient appears upset, it is your responsibility to pay attention and, if possible, provide some outlet or comfort.

References

1. Gelman, D. "The Thoughts That Wound." *Newsweek.* 9 January, 1989: 46-48.
2. Navarra, T. "Cardiopulmonary PT: Looking at the Whole Person." *Today's Student PT.* Thorofare: Slack, Inc., 1987.

Exercises

1. Have one student play an aged, testy and difficult but verbal patient and another play a therapist helping her do range of motion exercises with her arms.
2. What would you say to a patient who refuses to do her therapy because she claims the last time she did them the exercises left her in pain?
3. You arrive at a patient's room for a therapy session and find her writing a letter. What do you do or say?
4. As you enter an eight-year-old patient's room for his first therapy session, he begins to cry. What do you do?
5. Have a student play a patient who is complaining to a therapist about the general lack of attention he is getting from the staff. Act it out and discuss.
6. A patient begins crying because her husband never visits. How do you react?

7. A middle-aged male patient says angrily, "If I don't get out of this place, I'm gonna die here!" What might you say?

8. A young married woman, an outpatient, arrives for therapy with a black eye and bruises on her arms and face. Before you can say anything, she says she fell down the stairs. Do you pursue your suspicion that she has been beaten and, if so, how?

9. A 13-year-old patient only recently able to walk without a crutch says, "I walked five miles this morning." How might you react?

10. What questions might you pose for a patient who wants to assess her needs and progress? Consider the "What's It Worth?" technique.

11. What approach might you take with a patient who wants to assume a passive role in her therapy?

Study Questions

1. During a first meeting with a patient it
   a) is a good idea to state your name, title and the purpose of the session
   b) is not necessary if it seems the patient won't remember or understand, is not in the mood or is a child

2. A good therapist should
   a) be able to treat a patient no matter what the patient's personality
   b) give the patient to another therapist if there are personality conflicts that will significantly diminish the effectiveness of the therapy

3. Which is more effective in getting information from patients?
   a) questions that call for a yes or no answer because the therapist can focus the patient upon the most important issues
   b) questions that call for patients to express themselves in their own words because these answers will be more informative if analyzed thoughtfully

4. Which words would be more effective in getting your patient to open up?
   a) Do you have . . .
   b) Won't you . . .
   c) Can you . . .
   d) Please explain

5. Acknowledging a patient is a person
   a) may help to motivate the patient
   b) may strengthen the rapport between patient and therapist

c) both a and b

d) neither a nor b

6. If a therapist perceives a negative mood or attitude, the therapist should

   a) persist for as long as it takes to get the patient to reveal his or her true feelings because therapy will be ineffective otherwise

   b) Persist only as long as there is a real possibility that the patient will open up

7. By acknowledging a patient's apparently negative attitude, the therapist may invite the patient to vent

   a) tension

   b) anger

   c) fear

   d) none of these

   e) all of these

8. Talking about negative conditions that cannot be changed

   a) is pointless and depressing

   b) may be a way to vent, which may lead to communication on a more intimate level

9. Once the patient has described his or her problem and some of his or her feelings, a therapeutic plateau

   a) has been achieved

   b) may be achieved if you continue connecting

10. An example of a therapeutic plateau is

    a) relief for the patient because his or her struggle has been shared

    b) mustering the power to delve more deeply into emotional disturbances and set up goals to alleviate them

    c) both a and b

    d) neither a nor b

11. It is a good idea for a therapist to remain silent but attentive if

    a) the patient needs time to compose his or her thoughts

    b) the patient wants to watch TV

12. If your patient assumes a sick role and says, "I don't want to walk; I want you to push me in the wheelchair," a good response would be

    a) I wish someone would push me around in a wheel-chair all day

    b) you don't have to do anything you don't want to do

    c) I understand you may feel it's easier to ride in the wheelchair, but perhaps you are feeling uncomfortable with becoming more independent.

13. If a patient blurts out "I'm sick and tired of all this," you should
    a) tell him to control himself
    b) ask him to explain what he means
    c) tell him nothing ever gets solved by getting angry

14. Your patient says, "I threw up." A good response would be
    a) But you're OK now, right?
    b) Ugh! That's disgusting!
    c) When did you throw up? And what happened after that?

15. Your patient says, "I have a pain in my shoulder." Your first response would be
    a) How would you describe the pain?
    b) Did you take your pain medication?
    c) We all have good days and bad days.

16. A patient says, "I was supposed to ride in the rodeo. All my friends will be there." You respond:
    a) Don't think about that. Think about getting well first.
    b) Life deals some tough cards sometimes.
    c) You miss your friends.

17. The patient says, "I can't do these exercises." Your response should be:
    a) Sure you can.
    b) I wouldn't ask you to if I didn't think you could.
    c) You can't do these exercises?

18. In identifying a patient's significant statements, the therapist will
    a) be helped
    b) not be helped by knowing her history

CHAPTER III

Getting Through to Your Patients

Myron A. Lipkowitz, RP, MD

Initial Interview with the Patient

Before your first conversation with your new patient, there are some vital preparations that are in order. The room—your personal office or an examining room—and especially your personal appearance are extremely vital to getting the patient-therapist relationship off to a positive start.

Before seeing a patient, be sure that your personal appearance is perfect. Your grooming and personal cleanliness must be impeccable.

How Do You Stack Up?

To make sure you stack up try this checklist:
- shower or bathe daily
- use deodorant to eliminate body odor
- keep your teeth and breath clean
- hair should be trimmed, not wild, and squeaky clean
- keep nails trimmed and spotlessly scrubbed, and if polished, use clear polish or a subdued, pleasant color
- shoes should be polished or cleaned
- uniform or other clothing appropriate for your setting must be neat and a flamboyant color or style makeup should be minimal, so as not to attract undue attention
- if wearing aftershave or perfume, keep it very light

- do not wear an excessive amount of jewelry and be sure there are no sharp edges or points that could injure a patient
- always wash your hands between patients
- always wear a name badge; it is best to include your full name and title:

James McNamara, Physical Therapist

Sizing Up Your Patient

If possible, try to observe the patient prior to any conversation. Possibly you can observe him or her leaving the waiting area and coming into your office. A host of impressions can be readily apparent to the alert observer. Note the patient's general demeanor, gait, dress and grooming, style and affect.[2]

The Patient Sizes You Up

That moment of critical first contact cannot be retrieved after it occurs. There is nothing like a friendly smile and a firm handshake, if the patient is physically able, to give the impression of warmth and put the patient at ease. You must transmit a sense of genuine caring to the patient. Transferring a feeling of comfort to another individual without smothering him or her in the process is the essence of your profession. Anyone can be taught how to massage a sore muscle or apply a cold piece of equipment to a body part; a true therapist heals by combining learned skills with a caring attitude.

A Typical Opening

"Hello, Mrs. Adams, nice to see you." (Explain your role to the patient.) "I am Chris Morton, your (physical or occupational) therapist. Dr. Brennon has asked me to set up a course of therapy following the guidelines of his prescription. Our purpose at Town Physical Therapy is to find ways to lessen your discomfort using treatments, such as ultra-sound or heat. But most importantly, we want to help your body use its own healing powers to recoup all or as much of your former strength as possible.[3]

"If at any time you feel the therapy should be changed or feel that there may be something additional to help you, feel free to bring it up. If it is within the scope of the therapy ordered, I can modify your treatment. If not, then I will need to contact your doctor."

At first, it is best not to address the patient informally by his or first name. With most patients, the formality will quickly become unnecessary.

> ### Greet Your Patient Properly
>
> Don't hesitate to ask the patient what he or she prefers to be called—this may make a patient more comfortable. If a person says, "Everyone calls me 'Pambo,' " you can start a lively conversation about that and discover many aspects of your patient's personality.

Remember, Dale Carnegie tells us, "A person's name is to that person the sweetest and most important sound in any language."[9]

> ### Introduce Yourself Properly
>
> "I am Christopher Jones, your physical therapist. Please call me Chris." Not "I'm Chris, your therapist." Not "I'm (not saying your name at all) your therapist."

If your first patient contact occurs in a hospital, the script will change somewhat.

> ### Whenever You Enter a Patient's Room
>
> Knock first. If the curtain is pulled, always address the patient before entering this area of privacy. Introduce yourself, "Good morning. I'm Katie Smith, your occupational therapist. Are you Mrs. Raymond?" If there are visitors, "Are you a relative of Mrs. Raymond?"

If you are addressing more than one individual, direct your comments chiefly to the patient if he or she is alert and comprehending, or to the patient's representative if he or she is not. Also, occasionally glance at the others in the room to include them in your conversation.

Interviewing Techniques

Although we recognize that the patient interview is of paramount importance for effective practice, whether for a family practice physician or a therapist, very few of us consciously sharpen our skills once we assume our professional roles.

"Like many human basics—parenting, teaching, sex—interviewing is seldom taught, or studied, even by those who do it often."—Mack Lipkin, Jr.[4]

How many practicing health care professionals have you met who have had formal training in the techniques of interviewing, let alone had their performance observed and effectiveness critically analyzed? Fortunately, the importance of interviewing is being recognized and many programs now provide formal instruction in this area.

Imagine reading a book about skiing until you had memorized every detail and then being expected to go out to the slopes and negotiate a moderate downhill slope through several curves and land on your feet the first time. That would be a very unreasonable expectation. You would have to be led through each step from level ground, through a beginners' hill and gradually make a successful downhill run.

Likewise, just by reading this and other books or articles about interviewing you cannot be expected to become a perfectly effective interviewer. The educational system is changing to recognize the need to monitor closely and guide novice therapists to assure their eventual competence in this vital area.

Each interview must have structure, and certain functions must be accomplished during each interview. To be effective, each function must be performed well and all structural elements should be skillfully integrated.

Encourage Patients to Express Themselves

Allow your patients to speak uninterrupted for a reasonable time. Beckman and Frankel in their *Annals of Internal Medicine* article, "The Effect of Physician Behavior on the Collection of Data," observed physicians in opening interviews. They found that only 23% of patients were able to complete an opening statement without interrup-

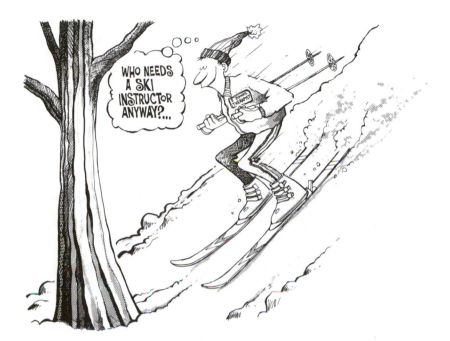

tion by the interviewer. They also found the average interruption occurred after only 18 seconds into the interview.[5]

Alfred Benjamin tells us in his book, *The Helping Interview*, that "beginning interviewers are often so concerned with what they will say next that they find it difficult to listen to and absorb what is being said.[1] Learn not to dominate the patient. Listen, because patients have something very important to say.

> Let your patients speak without jumping down their throats.

Communication Skills Improve with Maturity

New Jersey physical therapist Thomas Bartolino, after 12 years in private practice, tells us: "Communication skills improve with age, maturity and experience. It is an evolutionary process. You learn to have greater respect for the patient's desires. You become more subtle with time and more gentle. Physical as well as communicative skills become fine-tuned with time."

Bartolino's university training, like most, was very didactic. He was extremely nervous during his first personal contact with a patient. During his master's program, a course in interpersonal relationships began with a videotaped student-patient interview on the first day of class. Then, at the end of the course, it was compared with the first one. A great improvement in technique had been achieved.

Personal Warmth—An Invaluable Asset

Always greet someone with a smile; even a warm smile in a sad situation can be appropriate. How sad it is, for example, that a competent surgeon, although a genuinely caring and very nice person, never smiles when speaking with a patient. Many of his patients probably have said, "What a cold fish that Dr. Jenkins is."

Don't Be a "Cold Fish."
Try to appear relaxed and this will help an anxious patient to relax. When addressing or speaking to people, always look them in the eye, at least from time to time. Do not look at the ceiling, around the room or at the floor. Do not cover up your face with your hand.
Another important means of initial contact is the handshake. It is amazing how many people give a crushing or a limp handshake. People do judge you by such simple things. We may take it for granted, but many of us just don't consider the importance of a good handshake. If your patient is unable to shake hands, you may simply touch the patient's hand or shoulder.
Be friendly and courteous, but do not be overly friendly. Be careful not to let genuine concern be misinterpreted for a personal or intimate involvement. It is appropriate for a male therapist to acknowledge a pretty or pleasant smile, but it is wrong to say "You are beautiful." Also, avoid mentioning, "What a sexy perfume you have on," or, "Wow, do you smell good!"

Manner of Speaking

Avoid a monotonous tone when you speak, and while you may have to be somewhat authoritative, don't be a dictator. In other words, you may need to be firm but comforting.

Albert Mebrabian found that in delivering a message, over 50% of the process is nonverbal, transmitted through facial expressions and gestures. Less than 10% actually involves words. The balance consists of vocal tone, inflection and other sounds.[32]

While you should try to display optimism—even if your patient faces impossible odds—be as cheerful and uplifting as you can without making light of your patient's suffering.

If a patient has difficulty answering a question, do not rebuff him or her or otherwise imply that he or she is stupid. Try rephrasing the question.

If you are having difficulty getting a point across, try a diagram or written explanation.

Is the Patient a Hypochondriac?

Your patient was referred for a complaint of chest pain. You are providing him with therapy for arthritis of the spine. You know that the pain is radiating from this problem and is not angina (true cardiac pain). Because his left chest hurts, he understandably thinks he is having heart pain. You bring out a text that gives a table of causes of chest pain:—the most common sources of chest pain are the musculoskeletal structures of the neck, shoulders and thorax.[19]—it continues with a more detailed explanation should the patient care to read further. A WORD OF CAUTION—YOU MUST BE SURE THAT THE PHYSICIAN HAS INDICATED THAT THIS IS THE PATIENT'S DIAGNOSIS.

That a health problem is minor in your opinion but that you realize it is very distressing to the patient can sometimes be conveyed by saying: "Your problem is a major annoyance to you, and you seem out of sorts. Just remember that it's annoying, but it is not life-threatening. That is quite a difference."

Be cautious not to let the patient think you consider him or her to be a hypochondriac.

"Do you feel it's all in my head?" the patient asks. Your reply must be very carefully given to avoid conflict with the diagnosis provided by the referring physician. Tell the patient, "No matter what the source of your pain, my job is to give you relief by whatever modes of therapy your doctor ordered. Therefore, your doctor and I both believe that you are having pain and that it needs to be relieved."

Don't Be Judgmental

You can't expect your patients' values to be the same as yours. Do not be judgmental. You may be in a situation where you are providing services to a totally despicable character, possibly a rapist or a murderer. You must put your personal feelings aside no matter how difficult.

You may not feel you want to carry on a warm, overly friendly conversation with someone you strongly dislike, but, as Donna Ziarkowski, clinical assistant professor of physical therapy at the New Jersey College of Medicine and Dentistry, tells us, "There is no place for rude, abrupt behavior towards individuals. You have to put that thinking behind you. You simply cannot have that kind of behavior by a professional. If you don't like someone, just concentrate on the hand or the hip."

Ziarkowski goes on, "I once taught a prisoner how to walk following an injury, and one week later, I heard him mentioned on the six o'clock news. He had escaped. I felt like an accessory to the crime.

"Most often people will be nice to you if you are nice to them in a medical setting. No matter what kind of monster or felon they might be in the 'real world.' "

A Mix of Personalities

In a busy facility, a variety of personalities will be encountered. Be prepared to abruptly change the conversation if an embarrassing situation arises. An unthinking patient may start telling an ethnic joke, not realizing that the patient at the next table might consider himself the butt of the joke.

Be Realistic

When a patient is upset, try to put his or her problem in perspective. Emphasize the progress he or she has already made or is capable of accomplishing in the future. But it is equally important to be realistic and not set goals you know the patient is incapable of reaching, thus giving him or her false hope.

Patients Can Be Tough Questioners

How would you handle questions from patients or their families that require more thought than you can allocate at the time they are raised? Do not simply brush them off with a half answer or be rude and say, "I'm too busy for that now." Say, "Would you please be kind enough to write that question down (or call me later today or tomorrow) so that I can give your question the thought that it deserves?"

Or, "I understand your concerns, but I would appreciate some time to give you the correct answer rather than give you a rushed response—a rushed response that may leave you with other questions for which I wouldn't have the time to respond now."

If it is a difficult or complex question that requires some research on your part, do not be ashamed to admit, "That is an excellent question, but I'm afraid I'll have to research it and get back to you." Think how a patient might feel if you give a harried glance, and said, "I'm sorry but I'm too busy to answer questions now."

Being a Communicator

As broadcaster Barry Farber writes, "You and I have something in common. We both profit if we can get good conversations going and keep them going. What we don't have in common is what happens if we fail."

He goes on to say that his livelihood depends on his being a conversationalist and that his subjects may not know if they fail as such. "If you fail conversationally, your punishment may be unfelt and invisible. If I fail, I'm unemployed."[16]

Well, he certainly wasn't speaking to an occupational or physical therapist! If Farber fails he is the only one to directly pay the penalty.

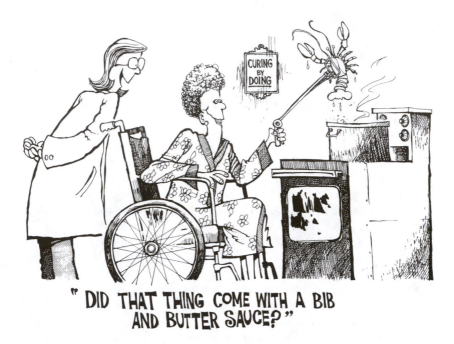

" DID THAT THING COME WITH A BIB
AND BUTTER SAUCE? "

If the therapist fails, his or her patient may pay the greater penalty. In the end, both suffer. It's a double loss. Farber goes on to say that as a broadcaster, his specialty is talk. His mission is to provoke conversations. Your task is certainly to try to get your patients to converse. If they don't open up and communicate with you, chances are your physical ministrations will be far less effective. When Farber's guests are articulate and cooperative, his job is easy. Many times our patients are unsure, nervous, ill at ease, frightened and in pain. Getting them to open up to a total stranger is a real challenge.

On a talk show, most subjects or guests certainly want to be there. While your patients may want to be in your office or clinic for your help, they would rather not have the need to be there. Some may actually be there against their wishes or even against their better judgment. They may feel they would rather remain disabled or unable to work. They may be unwilling to suffer the pain your therapy will bring. Perhaps they are malingerers and are not anxious to return to work.

"Communicating is something everyone does. It's as universal as eating, sleeping and loving, and as vital as any of these. Yet most of us do it so poorly so much of the time that we seem to discommunicate rather than communicate," wrote Philip Lesly.[22]

Roget's Thesauraus gives us examples of communicate and communication: to be in touch, be joined, converse, give, impart, inform, say, transfer, correspond, give information, letters, messages, social intercourse, speech, transference, two-way traffic.[10]

Two-way traffic! Keep that one in mind! It's a gem of an image.

> ### When we communicate, what are we really doing and how do we do it?
>
> —do we accomplish anything?—are we demanding?—are we editing what others wish us to convey?—are we confusing the issues?—do our methods cause disruption rather than healing?—do our petty personal objectives interfere in the treatment of the patient? Do we torment our patients with innuendos about other professionals out of professional jealousy?—are our words clear and concise? Do they get our message across or are they a jumble of technical jargon that goes right over the heads of our patients?

If you encounter a person of lesser intelligence, don't talk down to him or her. Your goal should be to use plain language, but not to make a patient feel stupid. It is amazing how often our so-called "dumb" patients simply have a lesser education than we do, but might have a higher I.Q.! They might never have heard a particular technical term but that does not mean that they cannot fully understand a reasonable explanation.

One doctor relates how she explained a difficult concept to a patient's husband, a mechanic. The patient had just had a difficult childbirth experience. "The surgery to suspend your wife's womb is similar to installing new shock absorbers," the doctor said.

"Hey, thanks, Doc," he replied, "that one I understand."

Most of us feel that when there is a breakdown in communications, it's the other person's fault.

Lesly added that the effects of discommunication are all around us. When parents can't understand why they think differently from their kids' thinking, it's called the generation gap. It's just another example of discommunicating. When husbands and wives discommunicate they often end up separated or divorced. And who could count the number of malpractice suits that are the result of discommunication?[23]

Lesly also wrote, "About 500 B.C. Confucius said: 'The whole end of speech is to be understood.' "[24] Using big words or technical jargon to impress our patients, will only confuse and frustrate them and is a mark of insecurity.[25] We should use language to close a gap between us, not to create a chasm.

That First Physical Contact

"First I would like you to put on this gown, so that I can examine you to determine the form of therapy most likely to help your condition. Do you have any questions at this time?"

"How long will it take before I am like new?" asks Mrs. Adams. "I have to get back to work. I have three little children at home."

"Let me make my assessment and then we'll discuss your situation and possibly I can answer some of your questions."

Topics of Conversation

During the course of the examination, light chatter about her children, job or other topic will generally put the patient at ease. Be friendly, but don't pry into personal matters. Remember to avoid discussing politics, religion and sex. You may insult, embarrass or anger your patient by discussing these issues. Of course, it is perfectly appropriate to discuss physical difficulties in performing sexual functions, if that is directly related to the reason for referral.

Personalizing Patient Teaching

Donna Ziarkowski feels it is helpful to know a patient's profession, vocation, education and other pertinent background. Ziarkowski said she would use that information to change the way things are explained to the patient, such as the terminology that is used. Ziarkowski might say to a patient who is not a therapist or physician, "Straighten or bend your finger." To another therapist or a physician patient, "Extend or flex your finger." Also, the approach to therapy would change depending on the physical level a patient needs to achieve to do his or her particular job.

Do Not Assume Prior Knowledge

Be careful not to assume that another health care professional who is a patient understands the principles behind a therapeutic modality. The benefits of a certain splint or brace should be explained to the cardiologist who is a patient or the automobile mechanic who is a patient, but the terminology you use might differ. While an orthopedic specialist who is a patient probably would need little or no explanation of his or her therapy or the purpose of a special splint, a cardiologist would probably expect a detailed explanation.

Undress Patients but Preserve Their Dignity

A prominent physician relates this story. A general practitioner in the coal-mining region of southwestern Pennsylvania noticed ulcerations on the tip of a women's fingers that suggested a rheumatoid disease. The patient was about 40 years old, had a high school education and seemed to have at least average intelligence. He referred the woman to a university-based internist for evaluation of this potentially serious medical problem. The patient returned to the general practitioner's office a few days after her visit to the specialist. "Would you believe that 'intern' you sent me to? She had the nerve to ask me to take my clothes off."
"Oh?" the doctor replied.
"Of course I didn't, I just walked out."
Then Dr. Lund called Dr. Ware, the specialist, and asked her what had happened. Before you assume Dr. Ware was just out of her residency and had no bedside manner, be assured that she was a fine and experienced physician with a very large practice.
Dr. Ware said, "I sat this woman down and took a history for about 10 minutes. Then I said, 'Let us go into the examining room and we'll get you gowned so I can examine you thoroughly.' With that she flew out of her seat and yelled, 'Who does he think I am, sending me to some "intern" who is gonna paw at me?'"
Realizing that even a wise and experienced professional such as Dr. Ware can at times have difficulty communicating with a patient, just imagine what obstacles the young therapist faces. This is a realistic confrontation. In a hospital setting, it usually becomes a nonissue by the time the therapist is involved. The impersonalization that many of us feel when put in a gown with our buttocks sticking out is usually accepted because everyone knows that's how it is. But in a private office, this can be a very sensitive problem.
What would you have done in that situation? Perhaps you could

say, "Although the only symptoms you are conscious of are the ulcerations on the tips of your fingers, your illness may be a type that can affect many different parts of the body. It is essential to examine your whole body, to search for small hemorrhages under the skin, to assess whether your liver or spleen is enlarged, check for internal bleeding with a rectal exam and so on."

If she still refuses, ask the patient if you might examine each extremity individually, especially her feet. Then examine as far as possible and gradually try to expand the exam with each visit.

Summarizing the Initial Examination

When the formal physical examination is completed recommendations are made and questions are answered. A straightforward, honest approach is the only acceptable one. Try to be brief and concise, but most important, explain in simple terms. For instance:

> "Mrs. Adams, your doctor has diagnosed your condition as a cervical sprain, commonly known as a 'whiplash' injury or neck sprain. Most people recover completely with appropriate therapy; you'll talk to your doctor about that. Your recovery, if nothing changes, will take approximately six weeks."

Continue the discussion about ways to help the patient with simple household or job chores. Avoid prejudging a patient's response. It is better to hedge on prognosis than be overly certain. You can say:

> "In most cases similar to yours, if there are no complicating medical problems, you should recover satisfactorily in about three months. Most important, we must be open and very frank about your treatment and progress. You must not hesitate to let me know if you are either not improving or getting worse. If friends and neighbors are critical of your treatment, which often occurs, have enough faith in your physician and me to ask questions."

Allow Time for a Patient's Questions

Tom Bartolino urges, "Give your patients 'air-time.' Listen and let the patients talk." In the past, Tom said, he used to dominate the conversation. Now he is an excellent listener.

The initial evaluation may last 45 to 60 minutes. Try to pinpoint and answer any questions at this time. In a private office this time can be best spent on introductions as opposed to simply throwing on a hot pack and beginning therapy. In a hospital setting the evaluation time may be impractical, but if time allows, it is very worthwhile.

Sometimes patients have to be led through a question and answer session. They may not think of questions until they are ready to leave, which disrupts your schedule, or even after they return home, causing you to spend time needlessly on the phone. By anticipating their queries you will save a great deal of time and have a better relationship right from the start.

There will be times when a patient can drive you to distraction with questions. The greater your skills as a communicator, the greater your chance of a successful therapy. The identical hands-on treatment by two diversely different therapists can have incredibly different results.

Effective communication results in: greater patient satisfaction increased compliance improved outcome[14]

Not Every Patient Gets Better

Not every problem will have a solution. No one therapist will get the best result with every patient. The sooner we learn this, the better off the patient and therapist will be. This will also lessen the stress levels of everyday living and working. It is wiser to remove yourself from an untenable situation early, rather than wait until it reaches a crisis point.

If a patient is fighting your attempts to treat him either physically or emotionally, confront him politely. "There seems to be a block in our progress. Do you agree that things have reached an obstacle that we can't seem to overcome?"

"What do you see as the problem?"

"What do you see as the solution?"

"Are you doing the exercises we have discussed at home?"

. "Is the therapy causing you more pain or discomfort than you can stand?"

> A maxim: "You cannot cure the world."

Patients Must Remember Instructions Before They Can Follow Them

Does your patient understand what you have explained or instructed? Ask him, "Would you please repeat (or demonstrate) that last point, so I can see if I explained it to you clearly?" Also give brief verbal instructions and see if the patient can repeat the instructions five minutes later.

The best way to ensure understanding and compliance is to give the patient a written instruction sheet. How many times does the patient leave your office and a short time later call and ask about something you had explained in great detail?

Perhaps part of the problem is that many times we subconsciously sort information. A prominent physician in a teaching hospital was hospitalized for chest pains. After several days he told the intern on his ward, "I finally realize why many patients do not follow instructions. I find myself hearing only what I want to hear. I am told to lose weight and start a carefully regimented exercise rehabilitation program. And what do I do? I am planning for my next skiing trip already. Thank goodness this is finally sinking into my thick skull."

Are We Tuned In to Our Patients?

Because of the long periods of direct therapist-patient contact, there may be an opportunity to fill a communication gap existing in the physician-patient communication. At least one study in a large primary care clinic showed that in less than half the visits made by a patient, the patient and the physician disagreed on the patient's chief problem.

Perhaps the greatest misunderstandings result from the busy physician's inability to grapple with patients' emotional responses to their serious illnesses or injuries. It most often is not for lack of caring, but because of time constraints.

A study at a leading Boston teaching hospital found that patients from lower socioeconomic groups seemed to disagree about basic aspects of their care more frequently than did patients from higher socioeconomic groups. Could this be a result of a deficiency in these patients' medical care?

It's interesting that for the most part, doctors assume they understand their patients' problems no matter what their social or economic standing.[15]

Is it any wonder there are so many complaints about medical care in this country when doctors, therapists and other professionals feel they are tuned in to their patients' every need and their patients often feel just the opposite is true?

There may be times when the patient will know of a procedure or modality that either benefited or worsened his or her condition in the past. Let the patient know he or she is in control, and if discomfort occurs, the treatment can be discussed to determine if the degree of discomfort is warranted. It is vitally important to document in the patient's chart if treatment was stopped and the reason, or if the patient refused treatment altogether.

What Makes an Adequate Therapist an Outstanding One?

A "holistic" or total-person approach toward your patient can transform an inadequate or barely adequate therapist into an outstanding one. Look at the patient as a whole person, not as a separate limb or other body part on which to concentrate your efforts.

Don't Be Afraid to Change and Grow

It's never too late to improve your approach to patients. Take therapist John Blake, for instance. A local physician had wondered for quite a while why some patients he referred disliked Blake so much. He seemed pleasant enough whenever he discussed patients on the phone or in person. One day, an office employee offered a tip on why patients were requesting a change in therapist. The physician had referred her husband to therapist Blake for severe lower back pain with sciatica. Blake badly frightened him by telling the patient there was a good chance he could become crippled for life because of his pinched nerve.

To be truthful, although it rarely occurs with good patient care, there is definitely a possibility of a poor outcome. But in the PT's attempt to be completely honest with the patient, and more likely, to protect himself from a malpractice situation, he unfairly frightened the patient.

He could have put it much more kindly by saying, "We have very high hopes that your therapy will greatly improve your back pain, and you will be able to function at a normal or near normal level if you follow my instructions and come regularly for therapy. There should be slow but steady progress. Please don't expect a miraculous recovery overnight. It will take time, patience and lots of effort on both of our parts. I must caution, however, that a very small percentage of patients, perhaps 1 in 100, may have their conditions worsened by therapy, resulting in permanent damage to the nerves in the back or the need for surgery." (It is essential to give a real statistic here, not an estimate, if such numbers are available. If statistics are not available, say, "A small number of patients.")

Once in a while, you have to frighten someone into having tests that he or she may otherwise refuse. But if a person is willing to undergo a necessary evaluation, why frighten him or her needlessly? On rare occasions, a patient will ask if he or she has cancer. Tell such a patient, "I'm sorry, but that is something to be discussed only with your doctor." You probably would wish to call the physician and let him or her know about the patient's inquiry so the issue can be addressed and the patient's anxiety relieved.

The physician involved in the above story about the therapist John Blake called and asked him out to lunch, and in a diplomatic fashion explained the proper approach in these situations. The therapist, instead of being resentful, was professional enough to accept this constructive criticism and changed his entire approach to these issues. Several days later the office assistant's husband returned to the therapist and could not believe the change in his attitude.

What If Advice Is Not Being Followed?

Sometimes a patient has to be told in no uncertain terms that a serious problem may exist. This is important, because if a person does not follow advice and has a serious complication or a more serious problem develops, he will often sue on the grounds that he was never informed about how serious his problem could be. He would argue that had he been told he might have cancer, he obviously would have agreed to all the tests he refused. Of course, it is the physician's responsibility to bring this to the patient's attention. It's your responsibility as the PT or OT to keep abreast of the patient's situation and communicate with him as therapeutically as possible.

Difficult Types of Patients

The Effects of a Patient's Cultural Background on Therapy

No two patients will react the same way to pain, illness or injury. You will encounter people with vast differences in their cultural, socioeconomic and ethnic backgrounds. Some may respond in a manner similar to how you would expect yourself or a member of your family to respond. Others may act in a manner totally alien to your concepts of so-called "normal behavior."

The relationship between the therapist and patient, depends on his or her recognition that attitudes toward pain may play a pivotal role in the ability to help patients.[50]

Although our bodies are similar, cultural influences in our lives cause us to deal with pain and suffering differently. We must work realistically with these differences if we wish to help our patients.[51]

It is important to note several points when dealing with ill or injured patients.

Some individuals will be very stoic and feel it is improper for them to admit to being in pain or that they are unable to perform certain physical tasks, such as walking or speaking. Others, with a relatively minor medical illness, physical deformity or injury will complain incessantly about pain or become depressed and difficult to deal with. These are opposite extremes and most patients will fall somewhere between them.

Also, be aware that some patients will demand a full explanation of the medical problem to the "nth" degree, while others will not request any information at all. In fact, some will be very upset about the details of their illness. Some will want assurances that they will be completely healed and will never have a similar problem in the future!

There are patients who refuse pain medication even though they are in great discomfort. Others cannot tolerate pain and want immediate relief. Even if strong narcotic analgesics are required, these individuals don't care about any potentially addicting properties or other adverse effects.[52]

Physical therapy can sometimes be very painful but necessary for recovery.

Overcoming Bias

No matter what our upbringing, most of us have been exposed to bigotry all our lives. Unfortunately, in some households and neighborhoods bigotry is not an undertone, but is blatantly expressed as a way of life. Perhaps there is latent bigotry in all of us. As professionals, most of us seem capable of keeping our true feelings suppressed, but unless we truly are as broad-minded as we would like others to believe, there will be times when our true feelings surface. Despite our good intentions, we must be on guard not to hurt the patients who may need us the most.

Take the therapist who is "color blind," in other words, one who wishes to treat patients the same regardless of their race or ethnic background.[26] By consciously ignoring the racial and socioeconomic differences between patients, we may be unable to accomplish our goals. Why? Because our patients may not be able to accept our values as theirs or our goals may be totally unrealistic for them.

Imagine an upper-middle-class patient deciding between taking a vacation or buying a new car and another patient from a poor neighborhood deciding, "Do I buy lunch or an extra few gallons of gasoline today?"

If you treat your patients of other races or ethnic groups with respect and are not condescending, you will be richly rewarded professionally, emotionally and spiritually. Your self-respect will also grow immensely.

The Angry Patient

Bigotry often finds its root in anger. How do you deal with an angry patient? The best idea is to allow the patient to vent his or her feelings. There is a phenomenon known as the "volcano effect." It takes about two minutes for the average person's anger to peak, the so-called volcano. Then, after reaching a boiling point, he or she will usually be reasonable. Therefore, if patients or fellow professionals get angry, let them have their say without interrupting. Each time a person is interrupted, the volcano effect will again start and take the full two minutes to build again.

No Pain No Gain

This phrase is seen hanging on the wall of many physical and occupational therapy facilities. It is on plaques and posters and handouts. Occupational and physical therapy may be very tedious. Both of these programs might be met with great resistance. They require all the patience and persuasive talents of the therapist to overcome this resistance.

Some patients have a level of anxiety that poses a greater problem than their physical disability. Anxiety may be a very real disability in its own way. Simply telling patients "it's all in your head" will not help them deal with these issues, but only worsen the problem. As was stressed earlier, if patients say they have pain, believe them; their pain is real to them. While you may feel that some patients are not that debilitated and are depriving others of your attention, remember they make up a significant percentage of most patient loads and if all your patients were the most severely disabled, you would be facing burnout very quickly. Also remember, if you make the effort, these patients will recognize your understanding and be a source of referral to other patients.

It is fully understandable that a patient whose livelihood depends on his or her strength and conditioning, and who is suffering severe back pain, will have a much greater anxiety level than a patient who generally performs only sedentary tasks. A white-collar worker may be more adversely affected by chronic headaches.

You can't change patients' attitudes toward pain and medical personnel overnight. Their entire lifetimes have been spent learning to respond to pain and other crises from their parents, older siblings and peers. Some patients will respond to you in the ways they feel are expected.

There are individuals whose skepticism interferes with your ability to help them. Others place an intuitive trust in their therapist and may be very badly hurt if their improvement does not meet their expectations. Caution is advised in handling both of these types. You must be as specific as possible with explanations of what they can realistically expect to gain by your therapy.

> MURPHY'S LAW: If something can go wrong, it will go wrong.

Do not demand blind faith in your abilities—"Murphy's Law" can always take over. We must protect ourselves as well as our patients.

Patients Most in Need of Communication Often Do Not Get It

Some surveys have found that as many as one of every four clinic visits were considered unsatisfactory because of communication barriers. In one such analysis, Korsch et al.[20] reveals that reasons given by patients were "lack of warmth and friendliness, failure to deal with the mother's concerns (for pediatric patients), use of medical jargon, and lack of clear-cut explanations concerning the diagnosis and origin of their illness."

It was evident that much more time is spent giving detailed explanations to a more affluent population, in other words, to those who

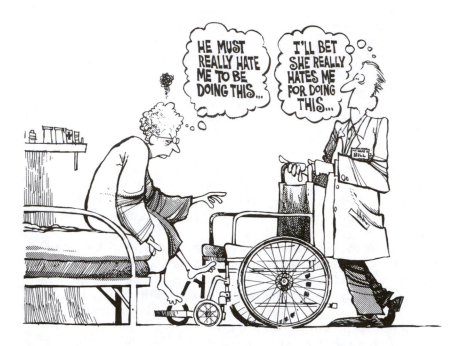

seem to be "more intelligent or better educated," in the opinion of the medical personnel. Those patients who needed more attention received less.[27].

Tips from Some Exceptional Therapists

Therapist Robin Pflieger, when confronted with a patient who is unwilling to put forth any effort, tries to motivate by "stressing the importance of the patient taking responsibility for his progress."

Ms. Pflieger boosts a patient's confidence by having him perform a task she knows he can do during the first visit, "even if he can only walk a few steps."

Beth Chack, supervisor of a head-injury unit, takes a realistic approach. She does not let failure to reach all of a patient's goals or her own goals for that patient get her down. She went into her profession knowing not everyone gets better. She asks her patients, "What are your goals?" during her first patient encounter.

"Some patients are overachievers. They must be restrained from hurting themselves by being so over-eager," says hospital-based therapist Jane Holloway. Others must be motivated by fear. "If they don't do it, they'll lose it. They have to be pushed," she adds.

"You can't be afraid to cause some pain during therapy," Holloway said. "If you are too timid, you can't do what is needed to help the patient and your kindness actually hinders or prevents progress. If this occurs it may be necessary for a more aggressive therapist to takeover."

Holloway makes an interesting point: "A patient may complain bitterly about being pushed and hurt by the therapist, only to be upset when on the therapist's day off, a covering PT or OT will not push as hard because of unfamiliarity with the patient's condition. Then the patient complains about this and compliments her regular therapist on her return. Very strong bonds develop between patient and therapist.

"Some patients who are touchy to deal with on their turf—their hospital room or home—will be easier to deal with on your turf—your therapy department or office, where they lose their security and you feel more secure," she says. Such an approach should be used with caution, however; don't be too intimidating. A patient's loss of security is certainly not your goal."

It is very important, Holloway says, that realistic goals are set by all parties involved, physician, therapist and patient.

"If a patient is not progressing well, but has gone to his limits, such as a patient with Parkinson's disease, there is no need to transfer him to another therapist. This may actually cause harm by giving the patient the sense that he can do better, when this is not realistic. Assure your patient that he has done very well and really achieved the goals set forth."

Holloway adds, however, that if realistic goals are not being met because of a therapist's inability to push that patient to his limits, it is time to switch to another therapist.

"Personality clashes are not always a reason to switch therapists, as long as the goals are being met," she says. "Many times a patient who was particularly difficult to deal with has come back weeks or months later and thanked the therapist for her persistence." Be more concerned about the patient doing well than whether the patient likes you.

Some patients need a structured approach if they are belligerent or disruptive, especially patients from a mental health unit. These patients have to be dealt with kindly but very firmly.

Your perspective changes after years of dealing with patients, and some hardening occurs. After dealing with a few quadraplegic patients you realize how much less significant are most patients' problems. However, one cannot lose perspective with other patients whose problems are very important to them.

Holloway believes you have to know something of each patient's history and physical limitations. "You can't always rely on a doctor's operative report," she says. The report may simply read "Patient is status post hip-pinning." That is not enough information for the therapist. What if this patient's osteoporosis is so severe that the surgical procedure was just barely possible? If there's any uncertainty, call the physician. He or she will appreciate it. After all, if that hip-pinning is not very secure because of the severe osteoporosis, and the hip disintegrates during aggressive physical therapy, both you and the physician will be held responsible. Lack of communication is no excuse.

"You must be creative; telling a patient he has to be able to transport himself 15 feet before discharge doesn't have as much meaning as, 'When you can get yourself from your bed to your bathroom at home, you'll be ready for discharge," Holloway says. "It might be just the motivation needed."

There are often great differences between what nurses will allow patients to do and what is going on in the rehab department. Everyone must read each other's notes in the chart. Example: a therapist saw a patient being lifted by four nurses and aides from bed to wheelchair. That same patient had been ambulating well without assistance the day before in rehab. Who knows why patients will allow that to happen? Some are senile, while others are just too timid to speak up against the authoritative nurse in charge.

"Many times, for various reasons, a patient will fail to give important information to his physician, often for selfish reasons, but the same patient may speak freely to his therapist," Holloway says. "It may be important to relay that information to the physician." Don't allow patients to make you promise not to tell the doctor.

She offers the example: a patient who is a heavy drinker, but who is afraid to tell the physician for fear he will be chastised or, even worse, refuse to continue caring for him. The therapist notices some trembling, an early sign of impending DTs (delirium tremens), a potentially life-threatening condition. Because of the bond with his therapist, the patient opens up about his drinking problem. The therapist then alerts the physician and preventive measures are instituted.

In this situation, the safety of the patient must override considerations for confidentiality.

You must be very cautious about prejudging patients. Therapists may be suspicious that back-pain patients are malingerers. You must not lose objectivity and sensitivity for your patients.

Manipulative patients can frustrate a therapist. Dorit Snow, an OT trained in Israel, was advancing very nicely with a dementia patient who had had a stroke, when her patient suddenly refused to cooperate. Snow discovered that the patient did not want to lose the assistance of her sister, who was doing everything, including feeding her. She insisted that she was being pushed too hard and wanted a different therapist.

Occupational therapist Lynn Jaffe realized it takes great ingenuity when dealing with "clumsy" children. Often, especially in the case of older children, they have already experienced so many failures that they either refuse to try a task, or give up if not successful after the first try. "I joke them through it," Jaffe says. "A lot of what I do is in a game form. At times I feel that there just has to be a way to get through to that child but I can't find it. I used to push harder and was very task-oriented. Now I have a much different approach and simply switch to a different format.

"Often I will tell a child of 9, who is having difficulty performing a task normal for a 6-year-old, that this is something usually reserved for 12-year-olds," she says, "thus building his confidence rather than tearing it down."

Depressed, Dying and Psychiatric Patients

The Grieving Patient

Among the most difficult challenges you will face as a therapist is helping patients through a period of grieving. Your patient may have lost a child, a parent, a spouse or other close friend or relative. His or her entire life may be changed. Yet he or she also may be in physical pain and require your services.

Sadness is something we all understand. We feel it when a personal tragedy occurs, but it can also be a symptom of depression. We become depressed when we suffer a serious illness, such as a stroke.

Usually our feelings of sadness and emptiness respond to time. Filling our lives with important chores may allow us to ignore these emotions. When this process is delayed, we may have to seek psychological counseling or even medications. It is the *unusual* delay that must be observed by the therapist and addressed in an appropriate manner. If the therapist cannot motivate the patient, the physician must be promptly informed.

However, great care must be taken not to interfere or mistake the normal grieving process for abnormal grieving. Our purpose here is not to detail at length this entire process; many articles and books are devoted to this subject. But a brief discussion is in order.

There are essentially three phases of grieving: (1) preoccupation with the lost person—mental conversations with the dead person and a sense of the deceased's presence, especially at night when the bereaved sees, hears or seems to be touched by the deceased; (2) disorganization—feelings of turmoil, emptiness, despair and contemplation of suicide, avoidance of social interchange; and (3) reorganization—finally a return to normal behavior and relationships. But, there may be sudden regression into either of the earlier stages by incidents that reopen the wound.[37,6]

The mourning process is very important. If it does not occur, it may lead to deep psychological injury later on. Signs of trouble include the inability to grieve immediately after a loss. Absence of weeping and prolonged hysterical behavior may be ominous signs; others include suppression of hostility that might be appropriate and self-destructive behavior, such as giving valuable possessions away.

Prolonged grieving may result in constant sadness, social isolation, generalized headaches, generalized aches and pains, or loss of the ability to function. Any of these signs indicates the need for intervention by a professional—a psychiatrist, psychologist or member of the clergy. It is essential that the therapist pick up on these subtle hints, because the patient may be far more open and feel less threatened by the therapist than by the family doctor.

Psychiatrists advise against using cliches such as "It's God's will," or "After all, you've got three other children," "At least you have the use of your arms," "Stop crying, life must go on." The presence of someone who quietly stands by, perhaps with a hand on the shoulder while the mourner weeps, is a comfort.[7]

Fear, Anxiety and Depression

When people are ill, they become depressed, anxious and cranky. Many patients' seeming hostility toward health care personnel arises from fear. The hostility becomes a defense mechanism. This should lessen after a few days and the fact that it does not may indicate that the patient has a personality disorder.

Excessive verbalizing, or the opposite—quiet withdrawn demeanor—are both signs of acute anxiety. Explanation and reassurance can be even more effective than medication for the anxious patient. Many patients have a preconceived notion of an illness. They may recall a stricken relative who never spoke or left the bed or wheelchair. They may falsely assume they are in the same position, despite a totally different prognosis because of modern advances, especially in the fields of physical and occupational therapy.

Even in hopeless situations, such as terminal cancer, concentrate your efforts on the positive. Say, "By continuing your therapy, we can hope to improve your strength to fight your illness and build up your tolerance to pain."

If you suspect a patient is depressed, you might ask, "How have your spirits been lately?" or "How have things been going for you lately?" Do not be surprised if you are greeted by an outburst of tears. The important thing is to be prepared to listen quietly while your patients unburden themselves. Be a good listener by just having patience. Sometimes patients just need a shoulder to cry on. Once they have opened themselves, there is a cleansing process that occurs in many, which alone may be very therapeutic. However, if you have the faintest inkling that the depression is serious, call the patient's physician as soon as possible.

If you feel the need to comment, you might say, "There is nothing unusual about feeling blue or down on yourself at a time like this. It would be very difficult to feel otherwise when faced with a prolonged or serious illness."[38]

You might say, "When you feel depressed or down about your condition, just remember that just a short while ago there was a question about your survival; now you are undergoing therapy. Therefore, you have already taken a very giant step forward. Now just keep taking one small step at a time, none of which are as overwhelming as what you have already been through."

Focus on the Future

It is important to focus on the plans for the future. Review the patient's treatment plan and set realistic goals. Even in cases where there may be little chance for rehabilitation of the body, there may be a chance for emotional response to therapy.

Post-Discharge Blues

Often, upon being discharged from the hospital, the patient feels a real letdown when he or she arrives home. The patient may be faced with enormous financial problems as well as difficulty performing the tasks necessary to survive. Even going to the toilet may be a difficult or impossible task without assistance. In the acute-care facility, help was only a button away; now there may be fear and anxiety—and a very demoralized person.

Minor aches and pains may become a great concern to the patient if located in an area of the body directly affected by a recent illness.

Things often ignored prior to hospitalization may now become a source of overwhelming fear to the patient.

Fatigue is a Forbidding Foe

After spending days, weeks or maybe even a month or more in bed, it is necessary to battle the atrophy of muscles and the sapping of strength that occurs. Therapists must constantly be aware of this and not let patients get caught in the web of fatigue. It means being persistent, no matter how much your patients insist they cannot continue and beg to be allowed to get back in bed. Your knowledge as a therapist must outweigh your feelings of empathy.

Fatigue often hinders recovery far beyond what would seem reasonable. Bedrest is the enemy. The effects of bedrest were dramatically illustrated by a study reported in *Circulation* in 1968, "of five healthy college students (three sedentary types and two trained athletes) who, after being tested in the laboratory, were placed on three weeks' bed-rest. Results indicated that the better the initial state of health, the longer it took to recover the original level of strength."[39]

The Dying Patient

Elisabeth Kübler-Ross is well-known for her work dealing with death and dying patients.

Her five stages experienced by the dying patient:

1. Shock and denial—initially denial may last anywhere from a few minutes to the rest of the patient's life. "No, not me!"
2. Anger—"Why me?" The frustration of the situation turns to outrage and bitterness.
3. Bargaining—"Yes, it is me, but ... " Patient puts a condition of acceptance on his or her illness, but hopes that he or she can live until a certain event, i.e., a family wedding, birth of a grandchild, etc.
4. Depression—"Yes, it is me." Weeping, brooding, despair and suicidal thoughts.
5. Acceptance—patient has worked out his losses and anticipates the end with quiet expectation.[40]

We must be careful to avoid trying to guide our patients through these stages. It is more beneficial to regard the process as normal reactions to any loss. The stages may appear in any sequence, simultaneously or disappear and reappear at any time.[40]

One important concept is competence in treating the patient. The greatest comfort comes from relieving the patient's physical problems. Another is compassion, which is derived from the Latin words *com* and *pati*, meaning to "suffer with." Patients can sense an attempt to fake this feeling. There is a grave misconception that we must be strong and not show our emotion when treating a patient. We are often taught to protect ourselves from emotional involvement with our patients. How wrong this is! We do not have to smother our patients with attention, but a show of true compassion for a person will never be forgotten.

Real involvement is not only unavoidable but necessary if we are to give our patients the therapy they need. Patients can be very quick to discern any pseudocaring and nothing infuriates a patient more than this perception.

In communicating with the dying patient, it is far more important to listen to the patient than to try to decide what to tell him or her. A patient might say, "I guess I won't need to save for a trip to Florida this winter." A poor listener might say nothing or, "Right. Don't worry about it." A better listener might say, "Why do you say that?" or "What do you mean?"[41]

It is important to develop conversation about the patient's accomplishments. Everyone has had interesting things happen during his or her lifetime. One therapist had a patient who seemed to be very cantankerous, until she discovered that he had been an officer at a military academy. His role involved ordering people around. She felt better then, knowing that she was not the subject of his demands, but that this was a way of life for this patient. By understanding him, she was in a better position to guide him through a difficult illness. Beneath his gruff exterior he actually had a warm spot or two.

Any member of the health team can help us appreciate the worth of any patient and can be a great influence on the outcome. Dr. M. had a patient for whom he had not developed any special feelings. Mrs. T. was dying from cancer and was developing contractures. Her physical therapist had developed a closeness with Mrs. T.; and as it turned out, they were from the same small town where she had been his high school guidance counselor. Instead of viewing her as just another shriveled-up patient, Dr. M. developed a very warm regard for her because she had been influential in the lives of one of the finest therapists with whom Dr. M. had worked. He realized that inside that fragile broken body was an intelligent and caring person.

Patients as Individuals

Don't refer to a patient as "that 80-year-old CVA," but as "Mrs. Bloom who has suffered a recent stroke." This applies whether a patient is terminal or not. Patients deserve and need a sense of importance. They do not wish to be "just another burden for the staff." If a patient has cancer, don't always assume he or she is terminal. One patient complained about a stay in the hospital where several health care providers—a nurse, a social worker and a student nurse—insisted on discussing the death and dying process with her. She became very assertive and told them she would most likely outlive them if they would just "shut up." She had a remission following radiation treatment and was still alive several years later.

Gentle humor has its place if the patient is coherent. I.G. was a patient dying of liver cancer a few years ago. He was in and out of a coma the last few days of his life. A few hours before his demise, he told his therapist a joke. As he strained in a whisper to relate his story, which could not be understood, the therapist thought how few of us die contented with life. It is, however, important to take your cue for humor from the patient, because an inappropriate humorous remark can be taken for callousness.

Alzheimer's Disease

Many therapists will be treating patients with Alzheimer's disease and other forms of dementia in their many stages. These are conditions of gradual and progressive overall deterioration. Motor skills diminish to the point of helplessness; patients will not recognize family members, much less their therapists. The disease can last for up to 20 years, although it generally averages 6 to 10 years. It is important to maintain body functions as long as possible, but this becomes an enormous task for both therapist and the family. Things seem worse in the face of hopelessness. It takes incredible patience to be kind to a person who is drooling all over you, or hitting and kicking and shouting at you.

Dementia is a group of symptoms related to a general decline in intellectual ability, severe enough to interfere with a person's ability to function normally. The patient is alert, but loses mental processes including mathematical skills, abstract thinking and judgment; speaking or coordination and changes in personality may occur. It differs from mental retardation, which begins at birth. Dementia is a change from a person's normal behavior.

Alzheimer's disease is only one type of dementia. Other causes are too numerous to list; but some of the more common ones are hypothyroidism, stroke, Parkinson's disease, brain tumors, medication and drugs. Opinions differ about alcohol as a cause. Studies have shown that Alzheimer's alone, or in combination with strokes, is responsible for about 70% of dementia cases.[28]

In the past, PTs and OTs were usually called in only if a patient's illness was considered reversible. Fortunately, this concept has changed and therapists are being called in early to help assess the patients' abilities to perform daily tasks and help maintain these levels of function if possible. Therefore, therapists are seeing many more of these patients, and an understanding of the complex nature of the dementia is important.[29]

One of the early difficulties with dementia patients is their denial and reluctance to admit that there is anything amiss. Early memory lapses may be covered up by long reminder lists. They tend to blame others for their mistakes. They will withdraw and shut themselves off from the outside world.[42]

While it is probably impossible to teach the patients new skills, it may be possible to teach them simple tasks if they are repeated often enough. An additional difficulty is the inability of a patient with Alzheimer's disease to process more than one thought at a time. The emotional processes go astray. Seemingly minor disturbances can appear to be catastrophic to these patients. They become overwhelmed with a feeling of hopelessness and being lost, a fear of strangers even though they are not being threatened by them. They may cry inconsolably, swear and use inappropriate language. It may be unbelievable to anyone who knew the individual in the former state. A person, for example, who used to bathe at least daily now refuses to bathe at all.[30]

Steps in coping and communicating:

—Remember, the person is not overacting "on purpose," the patient cannot help what he or she is doing.

—Take one step at a time. Reassure the person after each step.

—Reduce confusion by eliminating distracting noises, such as television, or a room full of other patients who may be well-meaning but boisterous and frightening to the patient.

—Be gentle and calm and don't overreact.

—Don't badger the patient with constant questioning.
—Don't force a patient into making decisions.
—If a patient is distressed, rocking, holding hands, patting or quiet music may calm him or her down.
—Do not argue or go into long explanations.
—Avoid restraining or using geri-chairs unless necessary to prevent them from injuring themselves, and then for as brief a period as possible.
—Take precautions so the patient does not wander off.
—You can recommended that the patient have an I.D. bracelet engraved with "memory-impaired," name, address and telephone number.
—If a patient undresses, give him or her a gown or robe or try to help him or her get dressed.
—If a patient makes sexual advances, distract with other activities.
—If a patient masturbates in an inappropriate place, distract or remove him or her to a place of privacy.
—If a patient is having hallucinations or delusions, try to convince him or her that the belief is incorrect, but avoid arguing.
—If the patient is frightened, quietly provide reassurance.
—Speak slowly and use simple, short expressions.
—Use a soft nonthreatening and friendly tone of voice.
—Be aware that Alzheimer's patients may mix up words, saying one thing but meaning something else.
—Discuss only one thing at a time; remember that the patient can only process one thought at a time.
—Also, be aware that an Alzheimer's patient cannot deal with abstract thoughts.
—Avoid questions that will only embarrass the patient when he or she may not be able to answer even simple ones.
—Avoid asking the patient to make choices.
—Use simple, direct statements: "It's time to eat" or "Go to the bathroom now."
—If the person uses offensive language, ignore it; do not take it personally.
—If you are accused of stealing from the patient, say, "I know you are upset because something is misplaced."[31]
MOST IMPORTANTLY, "DO NOT OVER-REACT!"

Often when a patient is faced with a serious illness, there is a regression to a childhood dependency on others. This can be beneficial if a person is hospitalized and if the dependency does not reach a ridiculous level. However, it must not lead to a degree of dependency that is so complete the patient makes no effort to help himself or herself. The therapist must strive to elicit the patient's inner strengths to help him or her heal.[47]

Mental Status Exam

PTs or OTs cannot pretend to practice psychiatry or psychology for legal and ethical reasons and, of course, because that is not their purpose. But their roles as therapists are so dependent upon their understanding a patient's psychological makeup that they must have a more than superficial understanding of psychological matters. Awareness of the mental status exam can be of great value.

Be certain patients do not feel belittled or that their intelligence is being questioned when assessing mental status. You might say, "There is a questionnaire that we complete for all our patients. It allows us to decide if there are any special techniques that will be necessary in therapy."

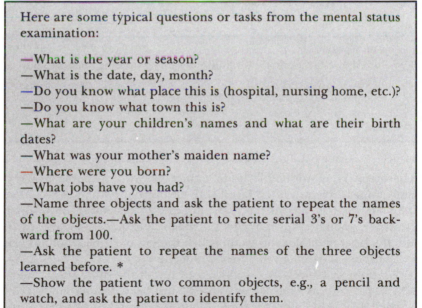

Here are some typical questions or tasks from the mental status examination:

—What is the year or season?
—What is the date, day, month?
—Do you know what place this is (hospital, nursing home, etc.)?
—Do you know what town this is?
—What are your children's names and what are their birth dates?
—What was your mother's maiden name?
—Where were you born?
—What jobs have you had?
—Name three objects and ask the patient to repeat the names of the objects.—Ask the patient to recite serial 3's or 7's backward from 100.
—Ask the patient to repeat the names of the three objects learned before. *
—Show the patient two common objects, e.g., a pencil and watch, and ask the patient to identify them.
—Ask about current events, a recent election, or storm or earth-

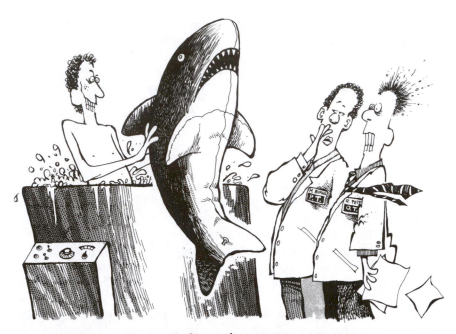

"FRANKLY, I'M JUST GLAD HE DECIDED TO LEAVE HIS HARPOON AT HOME ..."

quake, etc.
—Ask the patient to read and obey the following: "Close your eyes."
—Have the patient write a sentence.
—Ask the patient to copy a design.[43,8]

There can be considerable brain deficit before noticeable physical signs appear. We are often faced with an injured patient, who, other than the injured part of the body, appears to be physically normal. However, when therapy is begun, the patient's response is inappropriate. If a brief mental status exam is insufficient to provide an answer, the patient's physician must probe much deeper.

We must be especially careful not to forget the old axiom, "mentally ill patients also get sick or injured." Just because a patient carries a psychiatric label, never assume physical complaints are psychosomatic until they are proven to be so.

Communicating with Brain-Damaged or Emotionally Ill Patients

A paranoid patient may be very good at hiding his or her mental problems, unless provoked by a threat to his or her security. When dealing with a paranoid patient, it is important to spell out in detail every move or method of therapy, what he or she will feel and why it is being done. Although this should usually be the approach with every patient, it is especially necessary for these patients. Fear of being experimented on or harmed is characteristic of many brain-damaged and anxiety-ridden patients. Paranoia involves a distortion of the meaning of ordinary events. The patient's ability to assess things is impaired. If trust has not been developed between the therapist and patient, a vacuum of uncertainty becomes filled by the insecure patient's worst fears.

Mental Illness and Occupational Therapy's Roots

OT has been used for years for mentally as well as physically disabled persons. It enables patients to overcome or reduce their handicap and gain confidence in their ability to lead a normal or near-normal life.

Indeed, the origins of occupational therapy can be traced back to the late 1700s. Doctors, such as Philippe Pinel in France, Johann Christian Reil in Germany, and Benjamin Rush in Philadelphia, used OT in treating mentally ill patients. In fact, it is of historical interest that as early as A.D. 172, the renowned Greek physician Galen said, "Employment is nature's best medicine and essential to human happiness."

Rush, a highly controversial practitioner, was also a signer of the Declaration of Independence. Because of his communication skills, he was the most influential physician of his time. Despite his questionable practices of bloodletting and calomel purges, extreme even for his day, his efforts to improve the treatment for the mentally ill were humane and ahead of his time. By 1798, Rush had his patients being taught useful occupations, such as carpentry, shoe repair and needlework. Some even became musicians.[49]

Today's goals for occupational therapy have a much wider range, from basic functions, such as self-feeding and dressing, to useful ways to occupy time with games, crafts or exercise.

Innovation Improves Communication

Magician and illusionist David Copperfield created Project Magic, a group of volunteer magicians who train therapists to teach magic tricks to their patients as a means of therapy. Patients with little motivation are suddenly striving to learn more complex tricks as soon as they have successfully performed simple ones.

Imagine seeing a brain-injured patient, who might be very disruptive in a workshop, with his attention riveted to his therapist performing sleight of hand. A good example of this is a jumping rubber band trick, which strengthens fine motor function at the same time it holds the interest of the patient.

A surgeon, Dr. Neil Baum, studied magic while a college student to improve his fine motor skills. He now volunteers his time and is known to patients as "The Wiz." Dr. Baum stands before a group of his patients and says, "Sometimes you people may feel a little pulled apart like this newspaper," as he tears it in half. "Your fuse may be short, you may be frustrated." He tears it again and again. "But if you supply determination, hope and a little magic . . . , " Dr. Baum unfurls his newspaper, once again whole, ". . . then amazing things can happen to you."[46]

The Elderly

Many of your patients will be in the senior citizen age group—65 or older. Many of these "elderly" individuals are actually younger in body and spirit than people many years younger. Chronological age may not correspond to the body's condition.

Because of our lengthening life expectancy, between 1970 and 2025 the number of people older than 65 will more than double from 25 million to 51 million in the United States.[11] The goal of rehabilitation of the elderly is to restore independence. Dr. T. Franklin Williams, director of the National Institute on Aging, emphasizes the need for the nation to shift attention from acute care of older persons to continuity of care, which will maintain or maximize daily functioning so the elderly may continue to lead fulfilling lives.[48]

Age Not a Reason to Avoid Therapy

The following individuals have accomplished amazing achievements in their later years. They provide a marvelous example that age alone should not be considered a barrier to doing things with our lives.

Late, Great Achievers:

Konrad Adenauer (1876–1967) age 73–87, first Chancellor of the Federal Republic of Germany
Pope John XXIII (1881–1963), Pope at 77
Jomo Kenyatta (c.1894–1978), Kenya's first president at 70, for 14 years
Walter Hoving (b. 1897), chairman of Tiffany & Co. for 25 years, left to start his own design consulting firm at 84
Golda Meir (1898–1978), Prime Minister of Israel at 71, for 5 years
Dr. John Rock (b.1890), at 70 developed the birth control pill
Arthur Rubinstein (b.1897), at 89 gave one of his greatest concerts at Carnegie Hall
Frank Lloyd Wright (1869–1959) completed the design of the Guggenheim Museum at age 89 [12]

Psychologist Lawrence Casler of the State University College in Onesco, N.Y., is convinced that aging is entirely psychosomatic. In 1970, to break through "brainwashing" about lifespan, he gave hypnotic suggestion for long life to residents already 80 or older in a nursing home. Casler says that the suggestion appears to have reduced serious illness and added two years to the lifespan of those in the experimental group. Pollster George Gallop (b. 1901) tells us, "Intellectual curiosity is important, too. A lot of people die just from boredom. I devised a whole program that will keep me going until age 100 at least." Gallop performed a study of 450 persons older than 95, of which 150 were older than 100. He discovered that those who live a long time *want* to live a long time. They are full of curiosity, are very alert and "take life as it comes."[13]

In her book, *Activities and the Well Elderly*, Phyllis Foster tells us, " 'Old' is a state of mind that is largely dependent upon how one feels about oneself at any particular point in time and depends on mental attitude."

Everyone deals with age in his or her own way. Most of us consider that we will be old or elderly farther down the line.

Our elderly should be treasured for their wisdom, but unfortunately, many of our seniors are looked upon as burdens, felt to be "weak, dependent, senile, talkative, out of touch and closed-minded.

There seems to be a prejudice in our society towards aging and the aged. The victims of that social prejudice tend to believe those negative definitions of themselves and may very well accept and even expect the treatment they receive."[17]

While aging is not something that can be stopped or reversed, mental attitude about age can often be altered by positive thinking. Many people approach retirement with a very negative attitude, feeling that an end to their "useful" lives has arrived. They feel they are being "put out to pasture" until their will to live diminishes and they die. Their major goal is to avoid causing trouble to their families by getting sick or draining their finances.

A successful retirement should be approached as a new career. A time of opportunity to be anticipated, not feared. We must encourage our senior population to get involved in activities that will keep them healthy and feeling young. When our patients are injured or suffer a stroke, we have to convince them of the possibility of resuming a useful life.

One of the authors had a patient, let's call him Sam, who was a concentration camp inmate during World War II. Sam had suffered a stroke in his sixties, but despite a residual left-sided weakness, he continued to drive. He dragged himself around with a cane for about 15 years before he succumbed to a massive heart attack. Even during his last days, following the onset of his heart attack, he was a fighter. Although his heart was failing, Sam continued to maintain his spirit and drive and lived several days beyond medical expectations.

What can we learn from men such as Sam? That courage can often outplay the odds. Here was a man who suffered a stroke that for many would have meant putting a useful life to rest, even if they continued to live. But Sam lived a more active life despite his handicap than many retired people who are completely healthy. This is living proof that attitude can be a terrific stimulus.

We have to motivate our elderly. How many people do you know who do not act their age? The 89-year-old man chasing after women in his nursing home? The 35-year-old woman who has the blues and mopes around the house all day, who looks and acts as though she were in her sixties? We have to promote their sense of usefulness. Foster urges, "We must have expectations of our clients while allowing them opportunities to take risks. Life and living are risks! In this way, the older people we work with will be assisted in regaining and/ or maintaining feelings of dignity, self-worth, and their uniqueness as individuals." [18]

The Abused Patient

You must be very observant for evidence of an abused patient. If you notice that your patient has bruises, a black eye, or contusions that are not easily explained by an accident, you might suspect abuse. You may be dealing with a patient of any age. There are battered children, battered wives, husbands and the elderly.

You have a moral as well as legal obligation to report these patients to the proper authorities. Check with your state health department if you are uncertain of your legal standing in these matters.

Therapists are sometimes the only people these patients will confide in. You must keep an open mind and not be afraid to ask your patient questions.

Dealing with AIDS Patients

Acquired Immunodeficiency Syndrome (AIDS), was not recognized as a disease until 1981. By 1988, there had been more than 60,000 cases reported in the United States. Four groups of individuals account for the vast majority of cases: homosexual or bisexual men, heterosexual men and women who use intravenous drugs, recipients of transfusions, and hemophiliacs.

Persons with asymptomatic HIV (the virus causing AIDS) are capable of spreading the virus, and it is estimated that 20% to 30% of those infected will develop AIDS within five years. We can understand the fear associated with this dread disease when we are told that 80% of those afflicted are dead within three years of diagnosis.

We must remember, however, that health care workers are usually at no greater risk than the general public for catching the virus if they use common sense. In fact, those living in the same household with someone with AIDS, unless they are sex partners, are at virtually no risk of infection.

At last report, only three of 351 health care workers who had needle-stick exposure had developed the infection. There have been at least three cases of HIV infection after exposure of skin lesions or mucous membranes to infected blood.

Take into account that every transmission mentioned was the result of direct contact with contaminated blood. Therefore, the risk to an OT or PT is negligible, if it exists at all, unless the therapist belongs to one of the high-risk groups.

Feces, nasal secretions, sputum, sweat, tears, urine and vomitus, unless they contain visible contamination with blood, are not considered to be transmitters of the AIDS virus.[44] These are the most likely fluids that therapists will be in contact with during the performance of their duties.

It makes good sense to wear disposable gloves when touching any patient known to have or suspected to have AIDS or any infectious

condition. Patients are becoming accustomed to seeing gloves on
health care workers today. For instance, most dentists wear them with
every patient. It is important for therapists to refrain from patient
contact if the therapist has a contagious infection, such as a strep
throat, or a skin infection, such as impetigo.

It is important for us not to allow patients with AIDS to be made
to feel like the lepers of the past. The American College of Physicians
and the Infectious Diseases Society of America, as well as most state
licensing bureaus, believe that health care professionals are obligated
to provide competent and humane care to all patients, including
those with AIDS. The denial of appropriate care to patients for any
reason is unethical.[45]

We should approach AIDS patients like any other chronic patient,
not like a terminal case. Because of the possibility of a medical break-
through at any time, do not assume your patient will not live long
enough to benefit from your therapy.

Also, professionals must maintain the confidentiality of these patients, an ethic consistent with the duty to protect others and to protect the public health. Because of the unlikely possibility of spreading
AIDS through contact in a therapy setting, there is no need to put a
big sticker on an AIDS patient's chart or to keep those patients separated from the general treatment facilities used by other patients.

In short, when dealing with any patient, infectious or not, simple
common-sense precautions are all that is necessary. Above all, give
the patient the feeling that he or she is no different from any other
patient.

Helping Children Through Crises

Even a minor injury or illness will seem major to a child. Think
how this sounds to a child: "There is nothing to this operation to fix
your broken ankle. It's just a minor operation." To a child anything
requiring more than a Band-Aid is a big deal and can become a major
trauma to him or her medically and emotionally.

Dr. Sirgay Sanger, a noted child psychiatrist, tells us that children
under five often blame themselves for a serious illness or injury. They
feel that they must have done something terribly wrong to be pun-
ished in such a way.[33] They must be reassured that what happened is
an accident that could have happened to anyone.

Children often fantasize about an anticipated event and may feel
overwhelmed. They need to be carefully prepared. A mother or moth-
er-figure is essential to avoid a feeling of insecurity. It is a myth that

babies do not care who takes care of them as long as their physical needs are met.

You might tell them, "Even though you were unlucky and had an accident, you certainly are lucky to have a mother and father who care so much about you and such a good doctor or therapist to get you better."

The older child perhaps would dwell on "what might have been."[34]

After a traumatic event, such as a leg amputation, a child might revert to an earlier stage of development, such as bedwetting or day-time urinary or bowel accidents. Perhaps the child might develop a closer attachment to a parent or favorite stuffed animal. He or she may have eating problems, such as refusing certain types of foods or not eating at all. The therapist should be keenly aware of these diffi-culties and, if they are discovered by you before being apparent to the other team members, you can make a significant contribution by early recognition of them.

As soon as physically possible, the patient must be steered back to his or her pre-illness or pre-injury state of development. It is import-ant to prevent a pattern of prolonged abnormal behavior that may overshadow the original problem. Prompt attention to overcome ma-nipulative patients, whether child or adult, is a necessity.

Avoid judgmental remarks such as, "My goodness, son, what did you do to yourself?" [35] Instead, say, "I'm sorry to see you in that cast. Would you like to tell me what happened?" If he refuses, be patient and don't push. Usually the patient will open up to you if you don't seem too aggressive. Another approach would be, "I really would like to get to know you better. Then I can do a better job getting you back to normal. I can read your chart or ask your parents, but I would like to hear your ideas about what happened."

As a therapist, you may be attending to a young patient who has lost a parent or sibling in an accident. Avoiding discussion, or worse, hiding the fact, in most instances is not helpful. It is best that a person with experience dealing with these difficulties become involved from the onset.

The child who suffers the loss of a close one, such as a mother or playmate, should be encouraged to express his or her feelings from the time of the unfortunate event. The sooner this occurs, the sooner the mourning process proceeds through its stages and is eventually resolved. Reassurance of the parent's love must be reinforced. The parent did not choose to leave or desert the child.

We must remain aware that children will often blame themselves for the loss, especially of a mother. He'll recall his mother yelling, "How many times did I tell you not to leave your toys on the floor?

I'm so tired of picking up after you." Then, his mother fell asleep at the wheel and there was that terrible accident. His mother was killed, but he wasn't. He thinks, if only he hadn't made Mommy so tired! Repeatedly the child must be reminded that he had absolutely nothing to do with her death or serious injury.

The more difficult scenario is when a child's actions are the direct cause of a serious injury or death. For example, a mother drives into a telephone pole because she lost control while reprimanding her son for bad behavior. The crying and mourning must not be repressed. The pain will never be completely gone, but time does heal emotional as well as physical injuries. Repression may leave a person unable to come to grips with life for years.[36]

References

1. Benjamin, A. *The Helping Interview*, 3d ed. Boston: Houghton Mifflin Co., 1981.
2. Branch, W.T., et al. *Office Practice of Medicine*, 2d ed. Philadelphia: W.B. Saunders Co., 1987.
3. Branch, W.T., et al. *Office Practice of Medicine*, 2d ed. Philadelphia: W.B. Saunders Co., 1987.
4. Branch, W.T., et al. *Office Practice of Medicine*, 2d ed. Philadelphia: W.B. Saunders Co., 1987.
5. Branch, W.T., et al. *Office Practice of Medicine*, 2d ed. Philadelphia: W.B. Saunders Co., 1987.
6. Branch, W.T., et al. *Office Practice of Medicine*, 2d ed. Philadelphia: W.B. Saunders Co., 1987.
7. Branch, W.T., et al. *Office Practice of Medicine*, 2d ed. Philadelphia: W.B. Saunders Co., 1987.
8. Braunwald, E., et al. *Harrison's Principals of Internal Medicine*, 11th ed. New York: McGraw-Hill Book Co., 1987.
9. Carnegie, D. *How to Win Friends and Influence People*. New York: Simon and Schuster, 1981.
10. Chapman, R.L., Editor. *Roget's International Thesaurus*, 4th ed. New York: Harper and Row, 1977.
11. Coniff, R. "Living Longer." *Next Magazine*, May/June 1981.
12. Coniff, R. "Living Longer." *Next Magazine*, May/June 1981.
13. Coniff, R. "Living Longer." *Next Magazine*, May/June 1981.
14. Epstein, A.M., Taylor, W.C., Seage III, G.R. "Effects of Patients' Socioeconomic Status and Physicians' Training and Practice on Patient-Doctor Communication." *American Journal of Medicine*, 78:101, 1985.
15. Epstein, A.M., Taylor, W.C., Seage III, G.R. "Effects of Patients'

Socioeconomic Status and Physicians' Training and Practice on Patient-Doctor Communication." *American Journal of Medicine*, 78:101, 1985.

16. Farber, B. *Making People Talk*. New York: William Morrow and Co., 1897.

17. Foster, P.M., Editor. *Activities and the "Well Elderly."* New York: The Haworth Press, 1983.

18. Foster, P.M., Editor. *Activities and the "Well Elderly."* New York: The Haworth Press, 1983.

19. Friedman, H.H., Papper, S. *Problem-Oriented Medical Diagnosis*, 3d ed. Boston: Little, Brown and Co., 1983.

20. Korsch, B.M., Gozzi, E.K., Francis, V. *"Gaps in Doctor-Patient Communication." Pediatrics*, 42:855, 1968.

21. Kubler-Ross, E. *On Death and Dying*. New York: Collier Books, Macmillan Publishing Co., 1969.

22. Lesly, P. *How We Discommunicate*. New York: AMACOM, A Division of American Management Associations, 1979.

23. Lesly, P. *How We Discommunicate*. New York: AMACOM, A Division of American Management Associations, 1979.

24. Lesly, P. *How We Discommunicate*. New York: AMACOM, A Division of American Management Associations, 1979.

25. Lesly, P. *How We Discommunicate*. New York: AMACOM, A Division of American Management Associations, 1979.

26. Levy, D.R. "White Doctors and Black Patients: Influence of Race on the Doctor-Patient Relationship." *Pediatrics*, 75:640, 1985.

27. Levy, D.R. "White Doctors and Black Patients: Influence of Race on the Doctor-Patient Relationship." *Pediatrics*, 75:639, 1985.

28. Mace, N.L., Rabins, P.V. *The 36-Hour Day*. Baltimore: The John Hopkins University Press, 1981.

29. Mace, N.L., Rabins, P.V. *The 36-Hour Day*. Baltimore: The John Hopkins University Press, 1981.

30. Mace, N.L., Rabins, P.V. *The 36-Hour Day*. Baltimore: The John Hopkins University Press, 1981.

31. Mace, N.L., Rabins, P.V. *The 36-Hour Day*. Baltimore: The John Hopkins University Press, 1981.

32. Pease, A. *SIGNALS: How to Use Your Body Language for Power, Success and Love*. New York: Bantam Books, Inc., 1984.

33. Ramos, S. *Teaching Your Child to Cope with Crisis*. New York: David McKay Co., 1975.

34. Ramos, S. *Teaching Your Child to Cope with Crisis*. New York: David McKay Co., 1975.

35. Ramos, S. *Teaching Your Child to Cope with Crisis*. New York: David McKay Co., 1975.

36. Ramos, S. *Teaching Your Child to Cope with Crisis*. New York: David McKay Co., 1975.
37. Rubenstein, E. et al. *Scientific American Medicine*. New York: Scientific American, 1988.
38. Rubenstein, E., et al. *Scientific American Medicine*. New York: Scientific American, 1988.
39. Rubenstein, E., et al. *Scientific American Medicine*. New York: Scientific American, 1988.
40. Rubenstein, E. et al. *Scientific American Medicine*. New York: Scientific American, 1988.
41. Rubenstein, E. et al. *Scientific American Medicine*. New York: Scientific American, 1988.
42. Rubenstein, E., et al. *Scientific American Medicine*. New York: Scientific American, 1988.
43. Rubenstein, E., et al. *Scientific American Medicine*. New York: Scientific American, 1988.
44. Rubenstein, E., et al. *Scientific American Medicine*. New York: Scientific American, 1988.
45. Rubenstein, E., et al. *Scientific American Medicine*. New York: Scientific American, 1988.
46. Scheier, R. "Medicine's Journal." *American Medical News*, October 7, 1988.
47. Solomon, P., Patch, V.D., et al. *Handbook of Psychiatry*. Los Altos, Calif.: Lange Medical Publications, 1974.
48. Williams, T.F. and Jones, P.W. "Rehabilitation in Our Aging Society." *Aging—Special Issue on Rehabilitation*, 1985, no 350:2.
49. *World Book Encyclopedia*. Chicago: World Book Publishers, 1979, vol 14:488-9.
50. Zborowski, M. "The Effect of Culture on the Individual Cultural Components in Response to Pain." *Journal of Social Issues*, (8)4:16-30.
51. Zborowski, M. "The Effect of Culture on the Individual Cultural Components in Response to Pain." *Journal of Social Issues*, (8)4:43.
52. Zborowski, M. "The Effect of Culture on the Individual Cultural Components in Response to Pain." Journal of Social Issues, (8)4:45-48.

Exercises

1. Look at your self-portrait and list three or more things that you could do to improve your professional image.
2. What is the first thing you would say to a new patient? Is it appropriate or how could this first encounter be improved?

3. Looking back over your lifetime, list the three persons who have had a direct impact on your life. These can be a relative, teacher, member of the clergy, a close friend, or a boss whose ideals or examples you emulate. What are those ideals?

4. List three public figures, such as a politician, entertainer, sports figure, or professional person not known by you personally whose ideals you also admire. What is it that you feel is so special about them?

5. If you were to die today, for which qualities would you most like to be remembered? In one column, write all characteristics that apply to you now. In column two, write traits you would like to have.

Study Questions

1 By initially telling a patient to let you know if she is having difficulty in tolerating therapy at any time and that that therapy can be modified if necessary, you are
   a) putting the patient at ease and telling her that you expect to get important information from her
   b) making the patient ill at ease because you are not certain what kind of therapy program she should be getting

2. When a patient is in your office, it is important to respect his
   a) physical privacy
   b) the privacy of his records
   c) both
   d) neither

3. If you are speaking to a patient and a family member is present, it is usually appropriate to focus
   a) on the patient only
   b) on the family member only
   c) primarily on the patient but to occasionally acknowledge the family member's presence

4. During an initial patient appointment it is best
   a) for you to continually take charge of the conversation and elicit the necessary information
   b) provide a time for the patient to express himself freely

5. If your patient faces what appear to be impossible odds, your displaying optimism is
   a) phony and insincere
   b) still appropriate

6. If the patient asks for your opinion about the cause of his pain,
   a) you should avoid conflict with the physician's diagnosis
   b) you should not give an opinion
7. The problem with telling the patient the problem is all in his .head is
   a) he may feel you are discounting his pain
   b) he may feel you think he is stupid
   c) you are not giving him the information he needs to understand his problem
   d) he may choose to go to another professional who can help him to understand his condition
8. A patient is very distressed about a problem that is not at all a danger to her. You should
   a) reassure her but acknowledge her distress
   b) tell her not to worry
9. It is best to ask a patient of he has any new problems
   a) at the beginning of your appointment
   b) at the end of your appointment

CHAPTER IV

One Way to Spell Colleague is R-E-S-P-E-C-T

Myron A. Lipkowitz, RP, MD

Team Play

Physical and occupational therapists do not work in a vacuum! This means team play.

Who are members of the rehabilitation team?

—referring physician
—rehabilitation director
—physiatrist (specialist in physical medicine)
—physical therapist
—occupational therapist
—rehabilitation nurse (RN)
—social worker
—dietitian
—psychologist

Other health care personnel in auxiliary services or who interact in the health care facility:

—other registered nurse (RN)
—licensed practical nurse (LPN)
—nurse's aide
—pharmacist

—various custodial personnel

Physician specialties most likely to refer to a physical or occupational therapist:

—family or general practitioner
—internist (specialist in internal medicine)
—cardiologist (to cardiac rehabilitation programs)
—pulmonologist (to respiratory rehabilitation programs)
—orthopedist
—psychiatrist

Other health care practitioners with whom your patients may have contact:

—chiropractor
—biofeedback

Respect

Respect is something we have been taught by our parents and teachers since early childhood, for example: "Don't swipe another child's cookie," or "don't brush another child's crayons on the floor," "don't call someone naughty names." In its truest sense, respect means to hold in high esteem or honor.

> In our relationships with patients or colleagues, we often have to demonstrate respect without making judgments.

Respect in dealing with daily events should be a routine way of living. Being courteous, addressing an individual as Mrs. Jones, not as Helen, shows respect. You do not have to be in love with a person to demonstrate this respect. Simple acknowledgment of that person by his or her title may be all that is required.

Self-respect

Respect also means self-respect. It is difficult, if not impossible, to show respect for others if we do not have it for ourselves. If you have doubts about your abilities, these self-doubts lead to poor self-image and lack of respect for yourself. This will then project itself to your patients, colleagues and other professionals. How do you escape from this trap?

Look back and make a list of your accomplishments already. You have graduated from high school. You have been accepted into a health field course. Obviously somebody feels you have talent and intelligence and the will to be able to master the skills of physical or occupational therapy. You are presently involved in working and learning with other people in your profession. Physicians and nurses today realize you're a vital part of the medical team you are about to join. The vast majority of individuals in the health fields today not only respect PTs and OTs, but seek their contributions to the welfare of their patients. Patients have tremendous respect for their therapists, often giving them more credit for their outcome than the physician who prescribes it.

Trust

When a physician writes a prescription for therapy orders, physical or occupational, it reflects trust in the therapist. Let that relationship develop naturally and with time, that trust will build. The physician has the option of being very specific or very general in those orders. As an example, the physician can check the various individual modalities of therapy such as "ultrasound to the right shoulder" or simply "evaluate and treat." Often a bond will be formed between the physician and the therapist after they have worked frequently together. As the physician trusts the therapist's judgment, the "evaluate and treat" orders will become more frequent.

How does a therapist approach a referring physician when he or she feels there is a problem order? For instance, ultrasound is ordered for a teenager, but is contraindicated because the patient's epiphyseal plate has not yet matured to fusion. When more than 100 physicians were questioned in preparation for this book, the consensus was that physicians do not consider it a bother to receive pertinent phone calls from PTs or OTs about their patients.

What they do mind is failure to call them if there is a potential or actual problem and finding out from a third party, such as an attorney.

A physician learns to be a team player very early in his career. His function is to diagnose, plan, and prescribe treatment. He does not have time to spend hour after tedious hour with a single patient coaxing an arm to move or a body to walk. He knows a physician can't be all things to all patients. Similarly, a therapist must learn his role on the team and perform his function in relation to that role.

The following story is an example of importance of communication between therapist and physician in maintaining patient trust. George T., a physical therapist, was examining a patient referred for therapy for persistent hip pain. This hip problem, thought to be a chronic bursitis, had not responded to medical therapy as expected. George discovered a large lymph gland in the patient's groin adjacent to the involved limb. There were several things he might have done. He could have said to the patient, "Gee, did your doctor notice this?" Or worse, "I bet your doctor missed this. You had better go to another doctor who doesn't usually miss something like this."

What George did instead was to excuse himself and call the referring physician to inform him of this important new finding. In reality, he had been examined thoroughly by his internist, an orthopedic specialist, and by a chiropractor. This was not a previously missed finding, but a new development. The internist asked George to tell the patient that he had discovered something important enough to be immediately examined by her internist. The physician confirmed the findings.

Not only did the therapist preserve the patient's trust in her physician, but vastly enhanced his standing in the physician's eyes. The physician made it a point to stress how observant the therapist had been. One can only imagine the implications if the patient was led to believe the physician had "missed something." Fortunately there was a happy ending. Although this lymph node was the earliest sign of a malignancy, it was successfully treated and the hip pain was totally unrelated to this problem.

What were the aspects of respect in this matter? First, the therapist had enough self-respect and confidence in his abilities to take the proper course of action. He told the patient that a problem had arisen. Then he called the physician, who immediately spoke with the patient while she was still in the therapist's office. The physician had the patient come straight to his office, promptly saw her and complimented the therapist—in the patient's presence from his examining room phone—for this valuable and prompt finding. Everyone showed respect for each other. Both the therapist and the physician showed their respect for their patient by allowing her to know of the finding without hushed whispers behind her back.

Communication, whether between patient and therapist, therapist and therapist, doctor and therapist or between two other professionals, must have a single goal—to further the well-being of patients.

In a malpractice hearing, the term "misinterpret" or the phrase, "I

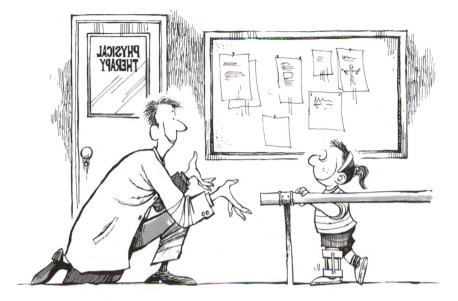

thought the doctor ordered something else," results in disaster for the defense. Communication must be precise and without ambiguity. If an order is not clear, call first. When calling the physician, do not blurt out, "I can't understand your order," or "You seem to have made a mistake." Use some discretion and common courtesy. You may well feel like saying, "What jerk wrote these orders?" Remember, you might misinterpret very clear orders someday and need that very same physician to back you up. A better way to put it is, "I am very sorry to disturb you, Dr. Miller, but I just would like to review your orders for Mrs. Smith. Would you mind going over them step by step to avoid misinterpreting your wishes?"

Relationships in the Work Environment

Health care facilities whether, private or public, are businesses. Many emulate large corporations such as GM or AT&T which spend thousands of dollars on programs to promote good will to the public and improve their image. The facilities accomplish this by working to improve the work environment and getting personnel to interact better, therefore projecting a better image to the public. If these programs were not successful, they would not be used year after year.

Many of us are familiar with Dale Carnegie's book and lecture series, "How to Win Friends and Influence People." His book has sold over 15,000,000 copies. There is no mystery about what he encourages us to do. If you sit down and make a list of things you can do to get people to like you, it shouldn't take long to realize that common sense and common decency are the roots of success.

One of Carnegie's "secrets" is showing a genuine interest in the other person. Most of us are interested in only "I," "myself," or "us." Listen to others and demonstrate your interest in another's point of view or their job and while you may not convert someone to your opinion, you will have a person who at least respects you and then be willing to listen to your side. Carnegie tells us that the only way to win an argument is to avoid one.[1]

Dealing with Inevitable Conflicts

Find something to compliment a possible adversary about and you will disarm him, before he has the opportunity to argue.

Betty, an OT, used to mumble under her breath every time one her student observers, Martha, asked a trivial question. The therapist's attitude abruptly changed towards her student following this comment from a patient: "Your student, Martha, certainly admires the way you care for me. She told me she considers you her role model."

There is a program called C.A.R.E. which hospitals use to improve the morale of staff and improve the facility's image to professionals, the public and patients. C.A.R.E. stands for courtesy, a positive attitude, respect, and enthusiasm.[2]

Those principles should be inherent to any health care institution, but we must constantly strive to maintain them. A positive attitude is needed by PTs and OTs everyday. We must leave our petty differences behind for the good of our patients.

No matter what your role is, a demonstration of human qualities will aid you not only in your relationships with other professionals, but with your patients as well. Personal and professional competence, human warmth, understanding, concern and a positive attitude are stressed by programs like C.A.R.E.[3]

In any situation where there are two or more persons with a common objective, there are bound to be conflicting opinions of ways to achieve their goals. We all have different expectations of life and this pervades everything we do. When we differ from our fellow professionals, we must find a common path to the benefit of our patients. We sometimes must compromise our ideals but must never compromise our ethics to the detriment of a patient. We must leave room for another person—fellow therapist, referring physician, nurse, or patient—to ease out of an uncomfortable stance. Don't push people to the limits. Confront a problem promptly before it gets out of hand.

If a problem or standoff arises, gather the party together for a conference. "Let's get our positions out on the table so that we can arrive at a solution to this patient's problem." The sooner this is done, the easier for everyone, and tensions will be at a lower peak.

Before jumping with both feet into any adverse situation, get the facts. Make a list of pros and cons.[4] Don't assume someone is against you before you hear an accusation. This situation arose a number of years ago. A long-time college friend, Harold, showed up one day in the clinic. He was passing through town and invited Bob B. to lunch. It just so happened he also noticed Jim S. working in the office. They had been acquaintances from high school days. Jim declined an invitation to join Bob and their mutual friend for lunch. Harold and Bob had a pleasant lunch and discussed good times past. The next day Bob left for vacation. Upon his return, he found that Jim had moved his things from the office they shared to a rear hall empty room.

Initially, Bob thought nothing of it, but finally he bumped into Jim and cheerfully wished him a good day. To his amazement, Jim glared at Bob and said, "You can't pick your relatives, but you can surely pick your friends." Abruptly Jim left Bob's presence. It was months before Bob could even get him to discuss the matter.

It seems Jim assumed that Bob and their mutual friend, Harold, spent their lunch discussing him in a derogatory way. Something very traumatic had happened to Jim during high school that was terribly embarrassing to him. In truth, Jim was not even mentioned, except for the friend to say that they had attended a prep school together. Not one negative thing was said.

Fortunately, because of Bob's persistence, Jim finally believed him and their friendship and trust resumed. But because Jim was not honest enough in his relationship with Bob, both individuals were deeply hurt by this misunderstanding and suffered for many months because of it. If they had been willing to discuss their problem, it would have been over almost instantly.

We must not allow hostility and negative feelings to become so distracting that they interfere in the care of patients. When a stressful situation occurs, try to find out the facts. Situations causing stress can be approached in a similar manner, whether dealing with a patient, or another professional. To a patient ringing for a nurse to remove a bedpan, five minutes seems like an eternity. To a nurse who has three buzzers going off at once, it seems like a very brief period.

Is a person being rude when he is getting it from all sides and has to make hurried and harried moves? How many of us in positions of responsibility carry our aggressiveness too far? There are times when aggressiveness is vital for the benefit of our patients. For instance, you are helping an obese patient get out of bed and she falls on top of you. There you both lie, unable to reach for a phone or buzzer, so you shout out at the top of your lungs, "Help!" Or, you are assisting a patient with a walker when the patient gets suddenly dizzy. You are worried that a fall would shatter her new prosthesis, and you yell out, "I need help, now!" In your situation this aggressiveness is comparable to the emergency-room physician yelling during a response to a code 99: "Get that I.V. going now! Give me those blood gas results STAT!"

At home or in the office, however, "Pass me the salt now!" or "Give me that chart STAT!" is not going to meet with much good humor. You have to remember where you are; you can't expect a great deal of tolerance of rude and inappropriate behavior. It grows old fast.

Problem solving phrases:

(1) "Tell me exactly what is happening."
(2) "When did you first notice this problem?"
(3) "Start at the top and give me a breakdown of everything that has happened to this point."
(4) "How do you feel we should resolve this issue?"

Useful phrases in stress situations:

(1) "I think I understand how you feel."
(2) "I can imagine how upset you are."
(3) "I can see that you're upset."
(4) "I'd feel the same way if I thought . . ."
(5) "I know it can be frustrating."
(6) "I think I've felt the same way myself."
(7) "I'm sorry you're upset." [5]

Once you've heard the other side of the story, it's best to clarify what has been said so far: "Let me repeat what you have said so far." Repeat what you have been told, pausing periodically for corrections or assurances that you have all the facts so far. Try to impress others with whom you're communicating that any solution is a joint decision which should be satisfying.

In any stress situation, above all, try to keep cool. Outwardly demonstrating your frustrations, anxiety, or dislike of an individual is not going to help the situation, but in some cases might turn a simple disagreement into a major battle. After a problem or stress situation is resolved, thank your former adversary for his help in formulating a solution.

In some situations, you may be the one at whose desk the "buck stops." If you are the boss, supervisor or other person in charge, you will have to face the music and make a decision. If you are caught up in a dispute but have the luxury of having a superior to consult, ask him or her for help.

Unfortunately, there will be times when you have to be tough, especially if you become aware that someone is clearly disregarding proper procedures. When society was less litigious, things were often allowed to slide because no obvious harm was done anyway. Today, that is not good enough.

Suppose a patient becomes dizzy and falls, but doesn't seem to be hurt. Upon being helped up, she says, "I'm so sorry I caused a fuss. I'm really not hurt." Everyone forgets it happened until a subpoena arrives requesting records of a fall in which your patient, Mrs. Smythe, was injured because of carelessness and recklessness of your facility.

Therapist A. was too lazy to make note of the fall in the patient's record. A note indicating that no apparent injury occurred should have been made at once. The physician should have been notified; it is his responsibility to put notes in the chart verifying his physical findings. The fact that no record is available will greatly jeopardize the case. It is clearly your responsibility in that situation to take action at once. First approach the person not taking appropriate action: "Gee, don't you think that you should record that incident in case there is a problem later on?"

"I don't have time; besides as you can see, she wasn't hurt."

Now comes the tough part for you, "Well, I have seen (or heard) of nightmare situations occurring just like this. My feeling is that it must be addressed right now and either one of us can do it. If you are too busy, let me do it and we'll both sleep better tonight. My gut feeling tells me to do it now."

If the other therapist does not agree, tell her you hate to go over her head, but you have no choice. By gradually working up to this point, in most situations, as soon as you've addressed the issue, the other individual would have agreed with the point you were making, eliminating the need to "go over her head."

Can you imagine the animosity that would have occurred had you promptly gone to your supervisor and said, "Did you know what happened in our department this morning . . . ?"

And remember this cardinal principle: Never argue in front of a patient or patient's representative.

In the introduction to his book, Philip Lesly mentions the common cry we hear almost daily to "bring people together" to "iron out their differences" and "to work things out." The remedy prescribed is better communication.[6]

Lesly tells us what happens when communications go astray. Most of us feel a breakdown in communications is the other guy's fault. But couldn't it just be that we sometimes fail to communicate?

Administrators get together, doctors hold executive committee meetings, businessmen hold board meetings, employees hold union rallies. How often do they get together with each other on a regular basis to establish good communications before disaster forces them to sit at opposite sides of the bargaining table?

Lesly wrote, "Each of us sees the effects of discommunication all around us. Parents and children discommunicate so much we have coined a term for it—the generation gap. Husbands and wives display their discommunication in the offices of marriage counselors and divorce lawyers. Employers measure their discommunication in turnover, absenteeism, and strikes. Doctors diagnose it in epidemics of pill popping, dissipation, government controls, and malpractice suits.

"Presidential candidates say simply, 'Trust me,' and find their biggest problem is in the public's distrust."

Perhaps people in health care should consider the impact of communication in the story of "mokusatsu." "Mokusatsu" is a Japanese word th. t can be used in two different ways. In one instance it means "to ignore," but it also means "to refrain from comment." Near the end of World War II, the Japanese made some overtures suggesting they might be willing to negotiate a settlement. A press release by our War Department used the word "mokusatsu" in the wrong context. Some historians believe the statement eroded communication between the U.S. and Japan to the point of prolonging the war and thus resulting in the bombing of Hiroshima and Nagasaki.[7]

If one word could tumble two nations, think of how vulnerable other people are to your words. In his book, *Professional Dominance— The Social Structure of Medical Care*, Elliot Friedson wrote that the professional's word is often assumed to be superior to that of the layman. After all, the professional is credited with having special knowledge and a noble, humanitarian heart. Why shouldn't his word reign over the layman's?

But should there be one segment of health professionals which dominates another? Friedson suggested "there are serious deficiencies in the nature of professionalism in general."[8]

Imagine what chaos there would be if there were no order in the health professional scheme. The physician writes a prescription for salsalate tablets for a patient's arthritis. This medication, although not too potent an anti-inflammatory agent, has no irritating properties to the patient's stomach. But the pharmacist decides to change it to indomethocin, a much more potent drug because he sees the patient is in such pain. The pharmacist does not know that the patient has a history of bleeding ulcers. Indomethocin can cause a great deal of stomach distress, even to the point of gastrointestinal hemorrhage. The patient would be exposed to a great risk if that switch were made. Therefore, by law, the pharmacist cannot change the medication prescribed by the physician without calling him first.

Another example would be the physician ordering physical therapy. His orders purposely omit hot-tub treatments for Millie Smith. Millie sees the hot tub in the therapist's office and asks if she might have that treatment added to her therapy for her bad back. The therapist says sure, not being aware that Millie's medication for her severe hypertension includes a potent vasodilator. A sudden severe drop in Millie's blood pressure could result in a stroke.

Now this does not mean that the physician should never be approached with a suggestion about treatment changes. Indeed, very frequently physicians will ask physical or occupational therapists for their evaluation and treatment recommendations because of the trust they have in the therapists' judgment. But this trust has to be earned.

There also has to be order in the care of a patient. Someone has to be the chief. Even among physicians, when several specialists are involved in the care of a complicated case, someone has to take charge, usually the primary care physician such as a family practitioner or internist, to coordinate the efforts in the patient's best interests. In this example it isn't the person with the most education, credentials or prestige. It is simply the person most likely to be in a position to represent the patient's best interests. Think of the internist calling a cardiologist to help in managing a complicated medical case in which a diabetic patient has had a heart attack. They both have similar but separate roles. They both monitor the blood pressure and heart rate and blood sugar. The cardiologist will order therapy according to the heart rate and blood pressure. The internist will, however, adjust the dose of insulin. The goal is the same for both; get the patient back on his feet.

Often there is competition among the therapists caring for a particular patient. Rutger's Professor Ziarkowski stresses in lectures to her students, that although there may be some overlap, PTs and OTs must learn to work together. OTs are more functionally oriented and PTs more physically oriented. With a team approach, the PT will put emphasis on being strong enough to do the chore and the OT will strive to help the patient perform it. Both therapists play a vital role.

Boston OT Lynn Jaffe put it well: "We have to have enough self-confidence that if someone else has a contribution to make, we are not going to feel threatened."

References

1. Carnegie, D. *How to Win Friends and Influence People*, New York: Simon and Schuster, 1981.
2. Friedson, E. *Professional Dominance—The Social Structure of Medical Care*, Atherton Press, Inc., 1970.
3. Lesly, P. *How We Discommunicate*, New York: AMACOM, (a division of American Management Associations), 1979.
4. *Managing C.A.R.E. Facilitator Manual*, Wheeling, IL : R.I. Gilberg and Associates, Inc.
5. *Managing C.A.R.E. Facilitator Manual*, Wheeling, IL : R.I. Gilberg and Associates, Inc.
6. *Managing C.A.R.E. Facilitator Manual*, Wheeling, IL : R.I. Gilberg and Associates, Inc.
7. *Managing C.A.R.E. Facilitator Manual*, Wheeling, IL : R.I. Gilberg and Associates, Inc.
8. Lesly, P. *How We Discommunicate*, New York: AMACOM, (a division of American Management Associations), 1979.

Exercises

1. Choose three members of the rehabilitation team, PT (if you are an OT) or OT (if you are a PT), referring physician and a staff nurse and describe their roles on the team.
2. In what areas of responsibility does your role overlap with these members of the team?
3. Do you feel that this overlapping is a problem for you to deal with?
4. If you feel that way, what do you think could be done to prevent conflicts with other members of the team?

CHAPTER V

Building and Keeping a Therapy Practice

Myron A. Lipkowitz, RP, MD

First Contact

"Each time employees confront customers, on the telephone or in person, they create a memorable impression of our service and our company. And this 'moment of truth' can determine whether the customer continues to do business with us—or leaves for a competitor."—G.R. Raymond, president, American Broadcasting Co.

Appointment Scheduling

Since PTs and OTs work in so many different practice settings and these may change many times during a career, you should be familiar with as many as possible. One of these is the small private practice. As mentioned in the quote above, a patient's initial contact with your practice makes a strong impression—for either better or worse.

Scheduling appointments can be very difficult. A patient who cannot be scheduled at a time that is convenient or prompt enough may be lost forever to a competitor.

Of course, a "no show" can be costly if a patient's allotted time was reserved exclusively for him or her, as may occur during an initial visit. Many surveys have shown that patients hate to wait. In fact, it may be the principle reason for being dissatisfied with a professional practice.

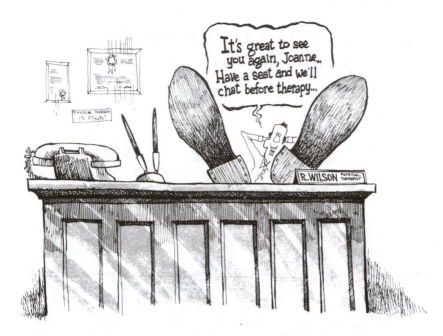

Information You Need from the Initial Phone Conversation

Whether a receptionist or the therapist answers the phone, the following information must be obtained: patient's full name, age, phone number—daytime and nighttime, who referred the patient diagnosis, if known by patient, or reason for referral, and does the patient have a prescription from the referring physician? Does the patient know what type of treatment the physician has ordered, type of insurance coverage, or who will be responsible for payment of services? Ask if the patient would like to know your fee schedule; if you require initial visit paid at time of services, inform the person at this time. The receptionist may wish to have a prepared standard "script"—questions you set up ahead of time—with a brief description of all or most of the services your facility offers, to answer simple questions. If the patient requests a type of therapy not on the list, the therapist should be asked if that service is available before scheduling it. This way, if the patient must be scheduled elsewhere, you will avoid wasting both the patient's time and your own.

There are two kinds of patients for whom scheduling is especially difficult. The first type is the demanding or abusive patient. These patients always seem unavailable when you have an open appointment. They assume that they are the only patient you have or that they are more important than others. They may actually have plenty of time on their hands, but they are used to being catered to.

> The demanding patient will call and demand an appointment at a particular time, as if he or she is your only patient. Such a patient feels that his or her importance outweighs any other consideration. People in this category are disruptive and manipulative. They refuse to believe other people have schedules, too. They may feel that this is the only way to get things done, or, simply, that they are important and nobody else counts. Not only do they demand a certain time, but when they arrive in the office, they want to be taken immediately and insist they have to be out by a certain time.

The second type of patient is very timid and may be suffering a great deal but not mention this on the phone when scheduling unless questioned.

An example: "Hello, this is Sally Holmes, I would like to make an appointment with your office."

Receptionist replies, "What is your problem?"

"I have pain in my neck."

"How long has it been there?"

"About six months."

"Well, let me see, we have our first opening on (a date three weeks from now)."

"Thank you. That will be fine."

What has not been communicated is: The pain has been present for six months, but since the night before, the pain has suddenly become severe and is radiating down the right arm, which suggests a pinched nerve or, at worst, a ruptured disk. This patient needs to be seen right away, or possibly referred back to her physician immediately.

It takes a very perceptive and highly interested receptionist to pick up on this type of situation on the phone, before you either lose a patient or the patient's medical condition deteriorates to become a further problem both medically and legally.

It should be standard practice for the person answering the phone to ask if anything has changed that would make the need for an appointment more urgent. It should be explained to the patient that emergencies arise daily and time must be kept open for such situations. Most important, if the patient cannot be accommodated, the therapist must make the final decision about when this patient is to be seen.

In some offices the final "Yes, squeeze them in," or "No, they can wait" can only be made by the therapist involved. Scheduling appropriately is essential for the success of any professional office.

There is an anecdote that dramatizes this point well. David, a dentist, ran into his friend Sam one day. Sam said, "It sure is nice to see you successful enough to be fully booked on a Wednesday when everyone expects a doctor to be on the golf course."

It seems Sam had an abscessed tooth and had called David's office Wednesday afternoon for an appointment and was turned down. David remembered that day particularly well, for he had left early because no patients were scheduled. After confronting his receptionist, Jane, he found out she had had something to do late that afternoon and did not wish to be late, so she arbitrarily did not book any appointments. It turned out that this had been a pattern of Jane's for several years. That means potentially thousands of dollars had been lost! His specialty was often needed on an emergency basis, and there were many other dentists in the area who were happy to see these patients.

Discussion of Professional Fees

Another sensitive area is the discussion of your professional fees. Here is a subject for total honesty. It is perfectly acceptable to discuss fees before beginning treatment. Actually, it is probably essential that you do so. Be prepared to defend your position, whether it be that payment is required at the time services are given or that you must be provided with insurance forms or some other commitment for payment. Be understanding but firm. If a patient mentions an inability to pay, then you have to search for the moral and ethical way to make arrangements with such a patient. Simply say, "We realize your predicament, but this office is not equipped to allow individualized billing. But we would be glad to accept a major credit card." This is an acceptable method of payment and most physicians, emergency rooms and other professionals accept them today.

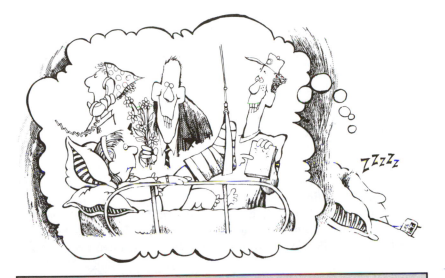

> **Physical Surroundings for Patient Encounters**
>
> Clean quiet, soundproof—eliminate distractions (radio, TV, beeper, etc.); well-lighted; private; avoid claustrophobic conditions (very tiny, closet-like room with no window, etc.); comfortable chairs and temperature; decor ranges from plain to luxurious depending on clientele; avoid clutter; don't leave confidential patient records and reports where they can be seen by others.

Remember Our Purpose

The Patient is of First Importance

The patient must feel as though he is the most important patient in your practice. At that moment, he must be made to feel as though he is the only patient you have. Avoid interruptions, especially during the initial encounter. Phone calls, knocks on the door, people who just want a word with you, secretaries who must have your signature at once, may well destroy in seconds what you have spent a considerable amount of time building. Obviously, you may have to make exceptions to being interrupted, but they should be carefully screened in advance. It is hard to put off a referring physician, but your spouse or children, or a patient dropping in for a signature on an insurance form should not be the cause of interruptions. However, a "Do Not Disturb" sign may be unnecessarily distressing to your patient.

Hurry Up and Wait

Nothing irritates patients more than to be kept waiting. Surveys generally agree that 20 minutes is the longest the average person will tolerate waiting without being upset. Whether it is your fault or not, the quickest way to get off to a bad start is to keep a patient waiting. Try to diffuse a patient's distress by immediately saying, "I'm really sorry I kept you waiting. I've just had one emergency after another." Or, "Something beyond my control detained me this morning and I wish to apologize for my delay." This almost always works.

If it does not, there is not much you can do except to keep these occurrences to a minimum. Despite your best efforts, should you find your appointments running late, try to prevent the rest of the schedule from lagging behind. One solution may be to change an appointment for later in the day to another time slot, which can get you back on schedule.

In a typical outpatient setting, 45 minutes is set aside for each initial evaluation, leaving a full 15 minutes for "overrun," phone calls, and so on before the next patient. It is a good idea to have patients fill out information forms before their time slots by asking them to arrive a little earlier.

What if the patient is late? When this occurs, you may explain: "We have a schedule to maintain and therefore we will need to cut your time short. But we will try to get everything in that is necessary to carry you through to your next appointment." Perhaps it is best just to make light of it and speed up your process, saying, "I realize you were late, but we'll do our best to get everything in that we do during an initial evaluation." Nothing changes between the two exchanges except your attitude, from annoyance—that the patient had the audacity to be late!—to your realizing he or she was late, but that it is important to accommodate the patient to the best of your ability.

When you begin, you can make a statement such as, "Let's get started so we can accomplish as much as possible during our 45-minute session."

Just when the therapist is closing a visit, a patient will often say, "Chris, I have another problem that I would like to discuss." This may become a major problem requiring more time to deal with than the original complaint. A way around this is to ask at the onset of each session, "What difficulties or problems do you want to deal with today?" Or, "Are there any new problems you wish to bring up today?" Then you can plan the visit accordingly, apportioning sufficient time to each problem by saying, "We will take one problem at a time, and if necessary, we'll schedule a follow-up visit."

Then, if the patient brings up something additional, you can say, "Well, ask Laurie at the front desk to give you another appointment as soon as it's convenient for you to deal with that problem."

Professional and Personal Ethics

It is important for patients to feel free to switch to another therapist if they are dissatisfied. They have a right to be aware of this and it is your duty to so inform them. Perhaps a small sign in your waiting area or in the examining rooms can be posted. Openness about this will be appreciated by patients and allow them to have a warmer feeling toward you. When it comes to professional and personal ethics, we tend to take our sense of values for granted, unless we are challenged by someone whose values are different.[1]

Daily we are bombarded with requests that challenge our ethics, morals and the law. A patient may say, "My attorney asked for another three therapy sessions so I can reach the 'verbal threshold' and then I can sue the insurance company for my auto accident." In many states, no-fault insurance laws allow suits only if a significant monetary damage amount is exceeded, thereby keeping many small accident claims from reaching the courts. A patient should not be kept in therapy merely to provide grounds for a law suit.

Or a patient may ask, "Can you give me a note for that day of work that I missed last month?" Your patient got up late and did not want to be tardy, so she called in sick, or told her employer she had to go for a physical therapy treatment.

It is very hard for most of us to say no. But millions of dollars are lost each year because of these "trivial" dishonest deeds. We must be firm and say no unless an excuse is truly legitimate.

A stock answer is: "I'm sorry, I sympathize with your problem, but I frequently get requests for a copy of our records to substantiate these seemingly minor excuses from employers and insurance companies and even school systems. Not only is it wrong, but if I falsify my records, or the chart does not substantiate the claim, I can be fined, or worse, lose my license to practice."

What a horrible penalty for such a "small" thing, but it really can occur. Beware!

How One Patient Perceived Her Therapy

The letter that follows was written to me. Chris Stonesifer, the patient, went to three physical therapists. All were registered PTs with many years' experience and were known to be competent and had busy practices. However, the results Chris got were vastly different. Why? Communication or lack of it!

Dear Doctor Lipkowitz: I have been to three different physical therapists. The first time for a shoulder problem. The therapists were OK.

The second time I went was for my chronic problem; it was a three-hour evaluation. I'd like to add that it was pure hell. The receptionist was extremely rude. The therapist had an OK personality. I felt extremely uncomfortable. The evaluation was carried too far in my opinion, because for three days after I couldn't move. He did not explain my condition; instead, he handed me a book on back pain and said read it, but you can't follow any of the advice in the book. Not too comforting. I was also told by this therapists' group, if I felt any pain at all, don't bother to show up.

A few months later I was in your office in excruciating pain. You sent me to see an orthopedic doctor, and he advised physical therapy. In view of my previous poor experience, I was reluctant to go. You recommended "Town Therapists." Jack S. is now my therapist. (Both names have been changed in the interest of privacy.)

They took me in quickly, even though I am a compensation case. I was extremely nervous and not trusting. "Town Therapy" and Jack S. were the best things that ever happened to me. The receptionist is kind, friendly and polite. I was made to feel very much at ease. Jack S. was very considerate of my feelings, he understood my mistrust, we talked and his honesty was very impressive. Any questions I had were answered and he explained that, "Yes, things sometimes would be uncomfortable," but I had to get past that phase of treatment in order to help my problems.

All the patients seem to be quite satisfied. It's as though the kindness they're getting they seem to give back. Anytime I'm feeling frustrated or down about the progress I'm making I can talk about it openly and honestly without feeling embarrassed or ashamed.

I would like to end by saying that I don't think I could be in more capable hands or get better care anywhere else. I have the best. You're treated as a person, not as an object.

Sincerely, Chris Stonesifer

(Mrs. Stonesifer of Howell, N.J., gave permission to use her real name as testimony to her strong feelings about her experience related to physical therapy.)

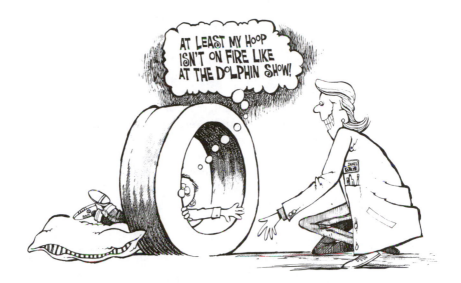

Above All Else, Remember the Patient

"A Patient" What is a patient? A patient is the most important person in our practice. A patient is not an interruption of our work; he or she is the purpose of it. A patient is not dependent upon us; we are dependent on him or her. We are not doing the patient a favor by serving him or her; the patient is doing us a favor by providing an opportunity to serve him or her. A patient is not an outsider in our business; he or she is our business. A patient is not a cold statistic; he or she is a flesh and blood human being, a human being with biases, prejudices, feelings and emotions like our own. A patient is not someone to argue with or match wits with, or try to outsmart; no one ever won an argument with a patient. A patient is a person who brings us his or her wants. It is our job to handle his or her requirements so pleasantly and so helpfully that the patient will return again.

Anonymous

References

1. Benjamin, A. *The Helping Interview,* 3d ed. Boston: Houghton Mifflin Co., 1981.

Exercises

1. Write a standard script for answering a phone call from a new patient requesting an appointment in a private office or clinic setting.
2. How would you handle a call from a patient known to be a malingerer, who requests an emergency visit when your appointment book is full for the next several days?
3. What would you say to a patient with whom you are not making the progress that should be expected in his or her situation?

Study Questions

1. When a patient calls and asks for an appointment at a time that has been booked solid, the call should be referred to the therapist
   a) always
   b) if the person taking the call is told it is an emergency or determines that it may be one after a thoughtful questioning of the patient
2. It is appropriate to discuss which of the following during the patient's initial phone call?
   1) diagnosis
   2) treatment sought
   3) fees
   4) insurance coverage
      a) 1 and 2 only
      b) 1, 2 and 4 only
      c) all of these

3. If a patient does not have insurance coverage, you
   a) must treat him and bill him for services rendered
   b) may require some type of payment at the time services are rendered

CHAPTER VI

A Lawyer's Approach

John G. Navarra Jr., Esq., JD

The Decision-Making Process

Before you begin to communicate with others, talk to yourself. You may discover quite a complicated person!

Your decision to become a PT or an OT should have been an informed one. Your studies have helped prepare you to make good decisions in treating your patients. As difficult as courses in school may sometimes seem as you are studying and preparing for tests, the challenges you will face when you begin working as a professional will be more difficult.

Each diagnosis and treatment will pertain to a unique patient, whom you may be encountering for the first time under serious circumstances. The patient may be afflicted by a number of conditions. He or she may be unappreciative, uncooperative and have bad breath. He or she will not be a patient in the abstract. You will be called upon to make numerous decisions for each patient you treat. How you go about making these decisions will determine how good a professional you will be.

In school you are given questions on tests for which you are to supply the "correct" answers. In your practice, when dealing with real problems, you will also have to ask the right questions of yourself, your patients and other professionals.

After listening carefully to the answers and assimilating the relevant information, you will more than likely formulate follow-up questions to clarify and confirm what you have been told. The memorization of facts will not be as important as understanding the information and knowing how to apply it appropriately.

Try to recall your thoughts at the time that you were making a career decision. That was, in a sense, your first professional decision. Jot down those thoughts and try to list them in the order of importance that you ascribed to them at the time.

How long did it take you to reach a final decision? To whom did you turn for guidance? How did you try to investigate your ideas? How soon after your decision to begin studying PT or OT did you make a commitment to yourself to complete your chosen program?

Was your decision an easy one, or were you considering a number of other options? What were they? Why did you not pursue them? What were the dominant factors influencing your choice?

These questions do not, of course, have any objective right or wrong answers. What is the right career choice for one person might be completely wrong for another. What is right for one patient might be completely wrong for another patient who has the same symptoms and diagnosis but different motivation, endurance, intelligence and family support. Choices about career and treatment alternatives should not be made without an appreciation of the individuals involved, their goals and their circumstances.

As a professional, your decisions will not be random; they will be based upon sound medical principles tailored to the needs of your patients. The difficulty will be in evaluating your patients and their conditions in a professional manner as you work through each step of their therapy with them. Effective communication is the backbone of that process. If you consistently make decisions in a professional manner, you should not run afoul of the law.

However, you may be sued during your career through no fault fault of your own. But just because you are sued does not mean you will be found liable or legally responsible. Our legal system provides for the peaceful settling of disputes. If someone believes he or she has been wronged, that person may sue. Perhaps the person (or persons) being sued is not responsible in any legal sense for the harm done. Perhaps no one is legally responsible. There should be no stigma attached to a person just because he or she has been sued. Being sued may be a stressful ordeal. The best way to diminish the likelihood that you will be sued at all, or that, if sued, you will be found liable, is to consistently make your decisions as a concerned, well-trained professional would. Effective communication is an essential element in that on-going process. Fine, you say. But how do I know if I am doing that?

Asking yourself that question shows that you are concerned about your professionalism. That concern should remain with you throughout all your years of practice. If it does, you will continue to grow from your experiences and will become better at what you do. Maintain a healthy curiosity and a desire to improve.

There is an old story about the farmer visited by a young scientist. The scientist promised to improve the farmer's techniques by advising him on the latest developments in agriculture. The farmer's response to the offer was: "No thanks, sonny. I don't farm half as good as I know how to already."

Having the knowledge is not enough. You have to be motivated to use what you know. That takes energy and attention to detail. Unlike that farmer, a health care professional recognizes a responsibility to keep up with the latest developments.

As a help to you in evaluating your decision-making skills, let's review your answers to the questions above about your first decision to become a PT or OT. Try to remember what you were thinking about when you first thought about these ideas, but also evaluate your answers from your present perspective. How has that perspective changed? How did you use communication in reaching your decision? How effective was it? Would you communicate more if you were making your decision now?

1. Over what period of time did you make your decision?
   a) one month or less b) six months or less c) one year or less d) more than one year

Unless you come from a family of PTs or OTs and were programmed from an early age to follow in their footsteps, there was a time when you did not know what you were going to do and a later period when you felt your course was charted. What you did or did not do during that time shows how you made an important decision.

There is no virtue in making important decisions more quickly than necessary. This is not to say a decision should be postponed for no reason.

During part of my career, I advised committees of business people charged with making decisions. Many of the committee members did not feel comfortable making decisions. Perhaps they did not have the intestinal fortitude they needed to take a stand. Or perhaps they did not have confidence they could make the correct decisions. It seemed to me we had two kinds of meetings—meetings in which the members claimed the decisions would be premature, and meetings in which it was too late to make and implement a decision for the present business year.

A decision should not be made until adequate information has been obtained. You should be thoughtful. Ask yourself, "What should

I know before I make this decision?" What should you know about a patient before you begin treating him or her? What are the contraindications for the treatment you contemplate? Are they present in this case? Does the patient have special limitations that will affect his or her participation in the treatment? Do your best to get the information you need, but realize that decisions must be timely to be effective.

> 2. Whom did you turn to for guidance? a) family members b) friends c) teachers d) professionals working in your field of interest e) no one

Some of you may not have felt the need to seek advice from anyone. Was this because you felt you had adequate information? Did you know you had adequate information then? Being a know-it-all is very risky. Did you fear that if you asked certain people they would have such definite points of view and be so persuasive they might lead you to a conclusion you didn't want to reach? Perhaps rather than risk that, you preferred not to seek their input at all.

You can learn to seek guidance and information from others without giving up your own professional independence. This is not easy at first, because you may be inclined to defer to their broader experience. Of course, you will want to be respectful of your superiors and consider carefully what they say. But you should not let your encounters with them suppress your own judgment and critical thinking. Learn how to express your concerns and questions in a diplomatic way that will show your concern and cause them to listen and take you seriously. You may be younger and less experienced, but you have been educated and you are a professional with legitimate concerns that should be respected. We will discuss later what to do if you are told to do something that you believe you should not do.

Did you discuss your decision with people who you felt would agree with you? Did this help to give you the confidence to make a decision at all? Did you use others as sounding boards to help focus your ideas? That can be very helpful.

If you spoke to many others because you didn't know what to do, did you substitute their judgment for yours? Was your choice really their decision at first? If it was, at what point did you make a personal commitment based upon your own experience and understanding?

Some of you may have felt it would show inadequacy to seek guidance from others. In all important decision-making, it is essential to get relevant, reliable opinions and information from competent sources. This does not show inadequacy. No one has a monopoly on truth. Recognizing that you do not know everything is a crucial first step in learning. Socrates taught that knowing that you don't know is the beginning of wisdom. Being willing to admit that you have more to learn and could use some help is an essential ingredient in any healthy professional life.

Do you recognize what you don't know? Do you know when you are not certain? How sure of yourself do you have to be before you make a decision to act? If the matter is of minor importance, you can afford to be casual. If the matter is very important, you should be as certain as possible. Especially early in your practice, it is a good idea to confirm each important decision by research and by discussing it with an experienced colleague. As you become more experienced, you will be able to judge more easily which decisions you are confident about and which require further consideration. How you make decisions will depend upon how clearly you think and how effectively you communicate. The quality of your decisions will determine the quality of treatment you give your patients and your professional reputation.

If you are given information by others, ask yourself if they are giving you their opinions rather than their objective observations. Can you tell the difference?

TABLE 6-1. HAZARDS ON THE ROAD

When you hear	Realize	Find out
I think or I believe or It seems to me...	You may be getting an opinion.	Is there a bias? Is the source an expert? What is the basis for the opinion?
He said or He told me...	You're getting secondhand info. or hearsay.	How reliable are the reporter and the original source? Can you verify the info.?
Let's...He should...She ought to...	You may be getting a conclusion. The speaker may be manipulative or directive.	For what purpose? To achieve what result? To avoid what problems?

TABLE 6-1. HAZARDS ON THE ROAD (continued)

I can't . . . Impossible . . . You can't . . .	You may be getting a conclusion. Your speaker may feel powerless and be seeking help or sympathy.	Does the speaker mean he doesn't want to or there is a difficulty and he would appreciate help overcoming it?
I need . . .	You are getting a conclusion. You may be hearing a plea or request.	Does the speaker really mean I want? For what purpose? What alternatives exist?
I will . . . We will . . .	The definiteness of the statement may mask that no basis for the prediction is given.	Is this a promise? By whom? Or is it merely a prediction which the speaker has no stake in? When "will" it happen? Is the prediction optimistic? Realistically so?
Always/never	You may be hearing an exaggeration used for emphasis.	Is the statement literally true? Is it really always or never? If not, is the patient exaggerating to show how severe the problem is?

I'm fine . . .	You may be hearing reflex answer or there may be an element of denial.	How does the patient feel in special areas of treatment or concern? Are there any new problems or experiences?

An observation is what the observer has personally felt, heard, seen, tasted or smelled. If someone gives an opinion, he or she is *interpreting* what he has observed, or, in some cases what someone else has observed.

Opinions can be useful, provided the opinion comes from someone who is competent to give it. If a person is giving you an opinion, is it based upon assumptions? What are those assumptions? Does it make sense to make those assumptions? Is the person jumping to conclusions and inviting you to join in? Failing to admit what you do not know and wanting to appear to know more than you actually court disaster.

> 3. How did you investigate the ideas you had about PT or OT? a) I mostly just thought about what I *thought* it would be like to be a health care professional. b) I just discussed my ideas with people who are not personally knowledgeable about the field. c) I discussed my ideas with guidance counselors. d) I visited a professional for several hours while he was working. e) I visited a number of professionals and observed them while they were working in different types of facilities.

A few of you may have felt you did not need to investigate your ideas very much. You may still feel that your education and what you have seen of your chosen field have not held many surprises for you. If you are among that group, you are rare, indeed. Most of us find that when we investigate our ideas, we gain new insights. These insights may lead us to change our minds. If they do not, they may well cause us to hold to the ideas we already had with renewed conviction and understanding.

What does this have to do with the law, you may ask. Some choose to view the law as a treacherous landscape that has been mined by unscrupulous lawyers and unappreciative patients. They believe that professionals must make their way through the landscape, which is so hazardous that many will be zapped through no fault of their own and no matter how careful they try to be. This is an unfortunate and very negative view. It is understandable that someone who feels he or she has been sued unjustly will feel wronged. But if he or she is to continue to function as a professional, he or she cannot afford to be so negative. That negativity will adversely affect your decision-making abilities as well as your relationships with patients and other professionals.

Although you may feel a sense of righteous indignation, you should not become so hurt that you resent the system and become suspicious of patients as the bringers of potential law suits. The best way to protect yourself is to be true to your commitment to the ideals of your profession.

Is your commitment an informed one? Were you aware ot the challenges, rewards and frustrations of the work when you made your decision? Are you inspired by the challenges? Are you content with the rewards? Do they motivate you to be your best self? Can you cope with the frustrations? If you can answer yes to these questions, you have an attitude that will guide you well.

You also have to ask yourself if you are being burnt out by the challenges and frustrations of your profession. If the challenges become drudgery, if the rewards seem inadequate and you feel cheated, and if the frustrations aggravate you on a daily basis, you will not be able to be the kind of professional you need to be. There is a danger that you will not meet the work's challenges. In such a frame of mind, you are more likely to take short cuts. You may convince yourself that what you are doing is not important. It is often the result of this kind of attitude that serious mistakes are made. What the law requires is that you act as a responsible professional.

4. How soon after your decision to begin studying did you make a commitment to complete your chosen program?
a) almost immediately b) within six weeks or less c) within six months or less d) more than six months

After you make a decision, do you feel you have to stick to it as a matter of pride?

Are you willing to re-evaluate your decisions as circumstances change or as you get more information? "Pride goeth before the fall" is a wise aphorism.

All decisions are in a sense tentative. It is appropriate to keep an open mind. Did you continue to evaluate your suitability for your chosen profession as you learned more about it? If you did, and your experiences confirmed your initial decision, then your commitment should be even deeper. You cannot afford to be inflexible in your treatment of patients; they are not textbook examples. Patients respond to your treatment in different ways. You should not make a decision about a course of treatment and be unwilling to modify it. Also, a good health care professional remains a lifelong student, continuing to learn and keeping up with the professional literature so as to do a better job.

Changing your mind or adjusting your course does not always mean you made a mistake. Even our best decisions are based upon available information. We rarely have the luxury of knowing everything we would like to know as we make and implement decisions. We do the best we can. As more information becomes available, we adjust or even take a completely new approach.

Evaluate your decision-making process. Did you communicate effectively to get the best information? Did you ask the right questions? Did you thoughtfully evaluate the answers?

If you do make an error, try to rectify it before it becomes a big mistake and significant harm results. Get the help you need from competent professionals. People will admire your candor and will be more likely to help you.

5. Was your decision an easy one?
6. Were you considering other career options? In what field? a) no b) another health care profession c) teaching d) psychology e) banking f) sales g) the military

If your decision was easy, was it easy because you were not allowing yourself to see all the possibilities that exist for you? What other fields could you have pursued? Was it an obvious choice because you knew yourself well enough and knew enough about the profession? Trying to see the possibilities is a challenge to your creativity. A really good therapist tries to see the possibilities for his or her patient as an individual.

How well do you know yourself? Have you ever taken a thoughtful inventory of your skills? What will it take to make you feel successful and fulfilled? What are your values? What do you want out of life? What are your goals? How consistent are they? Why would some of the other choices in question six not be right for you?

How easily do you get to know others? How well will you get to know your patients? How quickly and effectively can you introduce yourself, establish a trusting relationship and elicit the information you need without leaving your patient feeling as though he or she has been "processed"?

As you have reviewed the techniques in this book, you have become more skillful in communicating, but how you communicate should have the mark of your own personality. Do you feel at ease in your professional role? Can you make your patients feel at ease? Do you have a sense of what you need to do to be competent and effective? Do you make your job harder by setting unrealistic goals and feeling too responsible for others? Do you promise yourself and others too much? Do you needlessly make work for yourself?

The career options listed in question six require various types of communication skills. Yet there are similarities: Being a PT or an OT requires teaching skills. You are not only imparting information, you are also trying to explain how to do certain exercises to achieve maximum benefit and to avoid causing your patient further injury. You also may be teaching your patient to use an appliance.

An OT teaches daily life and self-care skills. He or she does not preach, but rather shows his students the possibilities that exist for them. The greatest achievement of the OT as teacher is to bring the student-patient to self-discovery and independence. With the therapist's help, the patient sees his or her limitations as challenges, is optimistic, and finds joy in meeting them. The patient comes to realize all of us have limitations and would rather strive to overcome them than be mired in self-pity.

> 7. What were the dominating factors that influenced your decision? The desire to/for: a) professional status b) heal/care for the sick c) money d) be closely involved with people e) be physically active f) have a challenging profession g) an easy job h) help people solve problems i) excitement j) please your family

It is a mistake to become a PT or OT if you are just looking for a way to make money. Would you really like to limit your practice to the rich, beautiful and healthy? Unless you anticipate significant satisfaction from helping others to become "better," healthier and more active, you probably should look for a different profession.

Some time ago, two friends of mine were in a similar situation; each had approximately $100,000 to invest. One decided to buy a house; the other used his money to start a landscaping business. Over the next seven years, the house on a waterfront property appreciated to a value far greater than the value of the landscaping business. The house owner gloated that he had made a better investment. The landscaper admitted that he wished his business were worth more, but he could not really be so disappointed. He had invested in a way of life, with challenges and rewards that he had found fulfilling day after day throughout the years.

Promises

Your patient needs your help and guidance. You are sensitive and feel compassion for her. You would like to alleviate the pain and rejuvenate the mind and body and make it better with a wave of a wand. You cannot. You offer no magic. You foresee no miracles. You promise to do your best. Even though you empathize, do not promise more than you can deliver. So much depends upon the patient. The patient must know and accept that. As the patient reveals her fears and hopes, you will want to reassure her. Therapeutic reassurance is an important part of your role. You should encourage your patient to hope for the the best, but do not promise specific results.

There are many reasons for this. You cannot be certain what the future holds for your patient. The results of therapy depend upon so many different factors. Imagine the disappointment of the patient who believes that a certain result will be achieved only to find that it will not be. Such disappointment will undermine the patient's confidence in you.

In some cases, juries have found that a specific promise amounted to a binding contract between the professional and the patient. When the specific result was not achieved, even though the professional had done nothing wrong, the professional was found responsible for failing to deliver the promised result. This is not the usual type of lawsuit brought by a patient. Most people recognize that you cannot promise, or warrant, specific results no matter how skillful and conscientious you are. However, if such a case is brought against you, it can be very detrimental, because professional liability insurance, also called malpractice insurance, usually does not cover a lawsuit for breach of contract.

What You Owe Your Patient

As you are treating a patient, you may become aware of personal matters that would be embarrassing or harmful to the patient if they were disclosed to others. You should respect and protect your patient's right of privacy. Law cases have held that unauthorized disclosure of medical records may be an invasion of the patient's privacy.

A special relationship exists between you and your patient. This is sometimes called a fiduciary relationship. Your patient has faith in your advice and treatment. In your fiduciary relationship the patient is particularly vulnerable to your influence, not just as it concerns treatment, but also as it concerns personal matters. You have a duty not to use that influence for your personal benefit to the detriment of your patient.

Accordingly, if you were to enter into a business arrangement with or to receive a significant gift from a patient, it could be claimed that you had used your influence improperly. In a lawsuit, it may well be your burden to prove that you had not taken unfair advantage of your position.

You should not seek gifts or tips. But what should you do if they are offered? Consider the spirit in which they are given. It would not be wrong to accept a token of gratitude on a special occasion. But what if the gifts are large or frequent? You should consider your patient and his circumstances. Is he really able to deal with his own affairs in a responsible way? Or are there others whom he relies upon? Do they know about the gifts? You must be scrupulously honest in answering these questions. It would be in the best interest of the patient and serve your professional integrity if you graciously explain that it is not ethical for health care professionals to accept gifts. Explain that you are paid, are glad to help and know that he appreciates your efforts. Be sensitive to his feelings and tell him that the offer will be remembered and is a gift in itself.

To protect the welfare of citizens, the law requires that health care providers must be duly able and careful. The legal principles and standards have been developed in cases dealing with physicians and surgeons. Many of those same principles and standards have been applied by courts in lawsuits claiming injuries caused by PTs and OTS.

It is your duty to use reasonable skill and care for the safety and well-being of your patient. You assume these obligations by becoming a health care professional. Failure to meet these obligations may constitute negligence. Negligence is defined in *Ballentine's Law Dictionary* as a lack of due diligence or care. Negligence is also sometimes called a wrong characterized by the absence of a positive intent to inflict injury but from which injury results, or a failure to perform a duty where the failure proximately causes injury to the plaintiff. The violation of a professional duty to act with reasonable care is called malpractice.

This is not to say that a professional must be perfect and that whenever an injury to a patient occurs the treating professional is liable, or legally responsible. Consider this case: A physician had performed an open reduction of a hip because of a fracture. Pins were used to unite the bones. Therapy consisted of abduction exercises and gait training. During one of the therapy sessions, the patient first walked through the parallel bars using a cane and then walked unaided by a cane, and then took several steps outside the bars unaided by a cane. The patient testified that the therapist was 15 feet away in a doorway talking to another person. The PT testified she was only about 5 feet from the patient. The physician testified that in his opinion the fracture was a stress or spontaneous fracture caused by a loss of calcium in the bone; so the break caused the fall and not the other way around. The jury was instructed by the judge that they should find the PT liable only if she had made a mistake that was inconsistent with the duty of care she owed the patient. The jury found no such mistake.

Caring professionals try to avoid all mistakes; but mistakes are made. Carefully consider each of the following examples. Which of them involve mistakes? The law requires a professional to possess and use a reasonable degree of learning, skill and experience ordinarily possessed by others of the profession. This is the professional's duty, which is owed to the patient. In which of the examples below do you believe this duty has been violated? Remember: Where the duty has been violated and injury has been caused by the violation, malpractice has been committed.

How might better communication and decision-making have avoided mistakes? Take notes as you read and think so that you can compare your ideas with those outlined below. The examples are incomplete fact patterns that are meant to raise questions as you read them. Make note of those questions as you consider each.

Examples

1. A PT administers ultrasound to a patient. Later it becomes known that there was a malignancy in the area of treatment. There was no mention of this in the report sent to the PT by the referring physician, but the patient did know about it and it was part of the patient's history taken by the physician's staff.

2. In administering ultrasound, the PT is filling in for another PT who had previously treated the patient. The substituting PT did not instruct the patient to report any uncomfortable sensation and the patient is burned.

3. A physician orders ultrasound to be administered to a 14-year-old boy. The PT questions the physician as to the contraindication because of the boy's age. The physician insists upon the

ultrasound. The PT complies, administering a negligible dosage. No apparent harm results.

4. A patent slides down from a tilt table and sustains hip injuries after complaining to the PT of feeling faint.
5. A patient falls and later complains that she was given inadequate instruction in the proper use of her crutches.
6. A PT gives a patient a new TENS machine without testing it or checking its setting. The patient takes it home, uses it and is burned.
7. Prior to hydrotherapy a patient complains of back pain. The patient's appendix ruptures and peritonitis results.
8. The therapist does not know that a patient is a diabetic. At the patient's request the therapist allows the patient to go in the hot tub without the authorization of the physician and the patient is burned.
9. The physician has prescribed therapy to ease the progression of contractures in an elderly patient. The patient complains of unbearable pain. The therapist stops the therapy and does not notify the physician until she calls to check on the patient's progress.
10. The patient arrives for therapy for tennis elbow and complains that he has chest pains, loose bowels and feels as though he is going to vomit. He says he has recently been treated by a physician for a stomach virus. The therapist tells the patient to lie down. During the next hour, the patient's distress intensifies and the therapist calls a taxi to take the patient home. The patient dies of a heart attack in the taxi.

Discussion

1. The report did not mention the malignancy. Was there anything in the report that would have caused a reasonably prudent PT to inquire further as to the patient's medical history? If there was and he did not inquire, he might be found negligent. Is it customary for a PT to accept and base the therapy solely upon such a report? Or is it customary for a prudent PT to also discuss the medical history with the patient? Did the physician prescribe ultrasound or did she simply order the PT to evaluate and treat the patient?
2. An understandable mistake is not necessarily a mistake that should be excused. Did the PT in this case act reasonably in assuming that the patient would be familiar with the procedure and know to report uncomfortable sensations? What is the pa-

tient's responsibility in remembering instructions previously given? What is the patient's age, health and level of intelligence?

3. What would constitute a negligible dosage in this case? How much time could pass before harm to the patient might be noticed? How is a therapist to react if he is directed to do something that he knows to be contrary to the welfare of the patient? He should speak to the physician directly, and tactfully and professionally express his point of view. If the physician insists that his order be carried out, and the therapist remains certain that the order is not proper, he should respectfully ask the physician to refer the patient to a different therapist.

4. Did the therapist take reasonable precautions given the patient's complaint? Or did the therapist discount the complaint? Did the patient cause or contribute to the accident?

5. What did the therapist do to instruct the patient? In patient teaching, the therapist must recognize any special difficulties the patient might have in mastering the skills being taught. Is the patient of limited intelligence? Does the patient have physical disabilities that hamper the performance of certain tasks? Did the therapist give the patient enough time to master the skills AND enough time to become comfortable with the skills? How did the therapist verify that the skills had been adequately assimilated?

6. What procedures are followed by the reasonably prudent therapist to determine whether appliances being used by the patient are safe? Does the therapist rely upon others to make determinations for him? How often are appliances checked? What are the risks involved in using an appliance? Is a patient adequately informed of risks?

7. Would a reasonably prudent therapist recognize back pain as referred pain symptomatic of appendicitis? If certain physical conditions are contraindications for therapy, does the reasonably skillful therapist have a duty to be able to recognize the signs of those conditions?

8. Why does the therapist not know the patient is a diabetic? Does a therapist have the authority to treat using therapy not authorized by the physician or might such activity constitute the unauthorized practice of medicine? Might such unauthorized practice be malpractice and expose the therapist to liability for any resulting harm?

9. A professional owes other professionals involved in a case the courtesy of keeping them aware of developments that they

might not otherwise know about. Has the therapist exceeded his authority in this case? Even if it was necessary to abate the therapy, would it not have been the duty of the therapist to contact the physician immediately? Would the therapist be liable for harm that might result from the suspension of the therapy?

10. By deciding that the patient is experiencing symptoms of a virus, is the therapist exceeding her authority by diagnosing? Would a reasonably skillful, prudent therapist have recognized a significant possibility that the complaints were symptomatic of heart trouble and secured competent medical care without delay?

Some physicians direct therapists to evaluate and treat. There is a difference between evaluation and diagnosis. Evaluation may involve the selection and level of treatment. Diagnosis is the determination of the condition existing and requiring treatment.

As you consider the above situations, you should realize they are examples meant to sharpen your sensitivity to the numerous circumstances that will challenge your commitment and skills. NOTHING IN THIS BOOK IS MEANT TO BE LEGAL ADVICE. You should maintain adequate professional liability insurance and be certain you comply with your responsibilities under your policy.

There can be no complete list of the varied situations that will confront you. The only way to prepare yourself is to sharpen your decision-making skills. They depend so much upon your ability to use what you have learned about your profession and effective communication. You must care enough to do your best.

Tips for Patient-Teaching

1. BE PATIENT. Remember it is not easy to learn something new even under the best of circumstances. How much more difficult for a patient who is sick or who has to cope with a new handicap? A smile and words of encouragement should reduce learning anxiety.
2. CREATE A RELAXED ATMOSPHERE. Distractions slow learning. Don't compete for your patient's attention.
3. GIVE SMALL BITES. Give your patient one idea at a time. This reduces confusion and misunderstanding and makes it less likely that all of a sudden the patient will be lost. Don't

be patronizing. Say you want to get it right and that's why you are going slowly.
4. REPEAT IMPORTANT IDEAS. Don't be boring. Think of different ways to reinforce what is important. Emphasize risks. Written instruction sheets are a good idea if they are well written.
5. LET THE PATIENT TALK. Draw the patient out. You will find out whether the patient understands and what her fears and questions are and you can address them.
6. VERIFY THE PATIENT'S UNDERSTANDING. Ask the patient questions. Have the patient demonstrate what he has learned by doing and talking.
7. DON'T LEAVE THE PATIENT ON HIS OR HER OWN UNTIL IT IS SAFE TO DO SO.

What the Law Requires of You

*ACT as an ordinary, *reasonable, skillful* professional would under the circumstances.
*SEE yourself as a professional inspired by the challenges of your work.
*REASONED decisions should precede action.
*MAKE decisions in a professional manner.
*BASE decisions on relevant, competent information.
*GET that information by using therapeutic communication techniques.
*DO NOT make unwarranted assumptions.
*SEPARATE opinion from fact.
*KEEP abreast of important developments in your profession.

Exercises

1. Why did you become a therapist? Was your decision easy or difficult? Why?
2. How do you plan to keep abreast of the latest developments in your field once you begin practicing?

3. What obligations must you fulfill under your state's law to maintain your license?

4. What should you know about a patient before you begin treatment? What will the sources of your information be? Are those sources reliable? How will you resolve conflicts in the information you receive?

5. To which professionals will you look for guidance? Do you respect and have confidence in those individuals?

6. Do you see yourself as a teacher? What types of teaching skills do you have in your inventory? How will you test your patients? Do role-playing in which you are teaching patients to use appliances of various types, do exercises, and so on.

7. Where do therapeutic reassurances end and imprudent promises begin?

8. Why is your relationship with your patient a fiduciary relationship? What is the significance of the term?

9. What are the hazards of taking gifts from or engaging in business dealings with your patients?

10. What is negligence? Is every mistake an example of negligence? What is malpractice?

11. Do you have malpractice insurance? Do you need it? How do you select an insurance company? Are you covered by an institution's policy? Does that policy cover all of your professional activity? What are your responsibilities under your policy? Does the policy exclude lawsuits for breach of contract? Are there other exclusions?

12. A therapist is being sued for malpractice. He wants to defend himself by claiming he was only following the referring physician's orders. What needs to be considered before it can be decided if that defense is a good one?

13. How should you react if a referring physician gives you an order that you believe is contraindicated?

14. What is the difference between diagnosis and patient evaluation?

Study Questions

1. A sweet, elderly patient of limited finances tries to tip you several dollars after a therapy session. You should a) take the money if she insists b) graciously explain you are glad to help and her offer is gratitude enough

2. If the therapist makes a mistake, that mistake constitutes malpractice a) always b) only if it is a mistake that a reasonably

prudent and skillful therapist would not have made and injury is caused by it

3. A therapist overhears a conversation between a patient and her daughter. If the therapist reports the contents of the conversation to the physician, the patient's privacy a) may have been violated if the conversation had no relevance to treatment b) has not been violated because the physician should be told everything

4. Each therapist a) should be covered by a malpractice insurance policy in his or her own name or as an employee of an institution that has a policy b) does not need insurance because the referring physician will be ultimately responsible for malpractice

5. If an accident occurs a) failure to contact the insurance company may jeopardize a therapist's coverage b) an attempt to settle responsibility in a friendly manner should be undertaken prior to reporting to the insurance company

6. Malpractice insurance is a) unnecessary if one is confident in one's ability and sense of responsibility b) essential because even if a therapist wins a malpractice suit, the suit still must be defended, usually at great expense, which cannot be recovered from the plaintiff

7. The standard of treatment the law requires a therapist to give patients a) remains constant and defined b) becomes more demanding as better methods are developed and as insights gained by the profession in general lead to individual therapists practicing their craft more skillfully

8. Which would constitute good therapeutic communication? a) I'll have you using that arm as good as new two months from today. Don't you worry. b) In most cases I've seen like this, excellent progress may be made in about two months. We can work hard together with that as our goal.

Appendix A

GLOSSARY OF LEGAL TERMS

CONTRIBUTORY NEGLIGENCE: A negligent act or failure to act which has helped cause an injury. A victim may have not been as careful as he should have been and may have been in part responsible for his injury. If a victim has been contributorily negligent, that may in part at least free the defendant of responsibility.

DUE DILIGENCE: A person must exercise reasonable care when he acts. How careful he or she must be depends upon the circumstances. When a professional is treating a patient, the professional must be duly diligent. That means he must use the skill and care that an ordinary professional would under the circumstances.

FIDUCIARY RELATIONSHIP: A fiduciary relationship exists between a therapist and her patient. This means there is a special confidence which the patient has in placing himself in the therapist's care. The therapist is required to live up to this confidence and trust by doing her best and by using due diligence.

LIABILITY: Legal responsibility. A therapist may be found legally liable for a failure to treat a patient as a reasonable therapist with ordinary skill would under the circumstances.

MALPRACTICE: An act of negligence committed by a professional.

MALPRACTICE INSURANCE: Insurance which covers the defense of malpractice claims and the payment of claims owed because of certain acts of negligence by professionals. You should be certain that the insurance you have covers you adequately in all situations where you work.

NEGLIGENCE: A failure to act as a reasonable person would under the circumstances.

PLAINTIFF: A person bringing a lawsuit to court. The person being sued is the defendant.

Suggested Readings

Activities and the "Well Elderly." Edited by Phyllis M. Foster. New York: The Haworth Press, 1983.

Ballentine, James A. Ballentine's Law Dictionary 3d. Rochester: The Lawyers Co-operative Publishing Company, 1969.

Beckman, H.B., and Frankel, R.M. "The Effect of Physician Behavior on the Collection of Data." Annuals of Internal Medicine 101 (1984).

Benjamin, Alfred. The Helping Interview 3rd. Boston: Houghton Mifflin Co., 1981.

Benner, Patricia, and Wrubel, Judith. "Caring Comes First." American Journal of Nursing 88 (1988).

Branch, W.T., et al. Office Practice of Medicine 2nd. Philadelphia: W.B. Saunders Co., 1987.

Carnegie, Dale. How to Win Friends and Influence People. New York: Simon and Schuster, 1981.

Clark, David G., and Blankenburg, William B. You & Media: Mass Communication and Society. San Francisco: Canfield Press, 1973.

Coniff, R. "Living Longer." Next Magazine, May/June 1981.

Darby, Patricia. Your Career in Physical Therapy. Englewood Cliffs: Julian Messner, A Division of Simon and Schuster, 1969.

Epstein, Arnold M.; Taylor, William C.; and Seage III, George R. "Effects of Patients' Socioeconomic Status and Physicians' Training and Practice on Patient-Doctor Communication." American Journal of Medicine 78 (1985).

Farber, Barry. Making People Talk. New York: William Morrow and Co., 1987.

Folstein, M.F., Folstein, S.E., McHugh, P.R. "Mini-Mental Status: A Practical Method for Grading the Cognitive State of Patients for the Clinician." Journal of Psychiatric Resident 12 (1975).

Friedman, H.H., and Papper, S. Problem-Oriented Medical Diagnosis 3rd. Boston: Little, Brown and Co., 1983.

Friedson, E. Professional Dominance—The Social Structure of Medical Care. Atherton Press, Inc., 1970.

Gazda, George M.; Childers, William C.; and Walters, Richard P. Interpersonal Communication: A Handbook for Health Professionals. Rock ville: Aspen Systems Corporation, 1982.

Gelman, David. "The Thoughts That Wound." Newsweek 9 January 1989.

Gilberg, R.L. and Associates, "Managing C.A.R.E. Facilitator Manual."

Wheeling: R.L. Gilberg and Associates, Inc. "Gracious Words." The Christian Science Monitor 25 January 1989.

Handbook of Psychiatry. Edited by Philip Solomon, M.D. and Vernon D. Patch, M.D. Los Altos: Lange Medical Publications, 1974.

Harrison's Principles of Internal Medicine 11th. Edited by Eugene Braunwald M.D., et al. New York: McGraw-Hill Book Co., 1987.

Hays, Joyce Samhammer, and Larson, Kenneth H. Interacting with Patients. New York: The Macmillan Company, 1963.

Johnson, Jerry A. Wellness: A Context for Living. Thorofare: Slack, Inc., 1986.

King, Mark; Novik, Larry; and Citrenbaum, Charles. Irresistible Communication: Creative Skills for the Health Professional. Philadelphia: W.B. Saunders Company, 1983.

Korsch, B.M.; Gozzi, E.K.; and Francis, V. "Gaps in Doctor-Patient Communication." Pediatrics 42 (1968).

Kübler-Ross, Elisabeth. On Death and Dying. New York: Collier Books, Macmillan Publishing Co, 1969.

Lesly, Philip. How We Discommunicate. New York: AMACOM, A Division of American Management Associations, 1979.

Levy, David R. "White Doctors and Black Patients: Influence of Race on the Doctor-Patient Relationship." Pediatrics 75 (1985).

Loughner, Phyllis, J. A Way to Survive—A Teaching Manual for Facilitating Alzheimer/Dementia Support Groups. Howell: Unpublished, 1988.

Mace, N.L., Rabins, P.V. The 36-Hour Day. Baltimore: The Johns Hopkins University Press, 1981.

Muldary, Thomas W. Interpersonal Relations for Health Professionals: A Social Skills Approach. New York: Macmillan Publishing Company, 1983.

Murray, Ruth Beckmann, and Huelskoetter, M. Marilyn Wilson. Psychiatric/Mental Health Nursing: Giving Emotional Care.

Navarra, Tova. "Cardiopulmonary PT: Looking at the Whole Person." Today's Student PT (1987).

"Physicians, Surgeons, Etc." American Jurisprudence 2d 61. New York: The Lawyers Co-operative Publishing Company, 1988.

Prosser, William L. The Handbook of the Law of Torts. St. Paul: West Publishing Co., 1971.

Purtilo, Ruth. Health Professional/Patient Interaction. Philadelphia: W.B. Saunders Company, 1984.

Ramos, S. Teaching Your Child to Cope with Crisis. New York: David McKay Co., 1975.

Robinson, Vera M. Humor & the Health Professions. Thorofare: Slack, Inc., 1977.

Rochester: The Lawyers Co-operative Publishing Company, 1973. "Why Physical Therapy?" American Physical Therapy Association. Washington, D.C., 1977.

Roget's International Thesaurus, Fourth Edition. Revised by Robert L. Chapman. New York: Harper & Row, 1977.

Science of Mind 61 (1988). Scientific American Medicine. Edited by Edward Rubenstein, M.D. et al. New York: Scientific American, Inc., 1988.

Scheier, R. "Medicine's Journal." American Medical News 7 October 1988.

Seymour, Peter. I Am My Brother. Kansas City: Hallmark Cards, Inc., 1972.

Smith, Voncile M., and Bass, Thelma A. Communication for Health Professionals. New York: J.B. Lippincott Company,1979.

Tonn, Joan C. Understanding the Other Person: Skillful Interpersonal Communication. Wellesley Hills: Educational Planning Services Corpo ration, 1985.

Weeks, Ruby B. "Liability for Injuries or Death Resulting from Physical Therapy." American Law Reports 3d 53.

Williams, T.F., and Jones, P.W. "Rehabilitation in Our Aging Society." Aging—Special Issue on Rehabilitation 350 (1985).

"Physical Therapy" and "Occupational Therapy." World Book Encyclopedia 14 and 15. Chicago: World Book—Childcraft International, Inc., 1979.

Xanthes. Speech: How to Use It Effectively. New York: Funk & Wagnalls Company, 1916.

Yoritomo-Tashi. Timidity: How to Overcome It. New York: Funk & Wagnalls Company, 1916.

Young, Edward. Night Thoughts. Boston: Lewis Sampson, 1842.

Zborowski, Mark. "The Effect of Culture of the Individual—Cultural Components in Response to Pain." The Journal of Social Issues VIII:4 (1953).

Index